Stefan Suwelack

Real-time Biomechanical Modeling for Intraoperative Soft Tissue Registration

Real-time Biomechanical Modeling for Intraoperative Soft Tissue Registration

by

Stefan Suwelack

KIT Scientific Publishing

Dissertation, Karlsruher Institut für Technologie (KIT)
Fakultät für Informatik, 2014

Tag der mündlichen Prüfung: 01. Juli 2014
Hauptreferent: Prof. R. Dillmann
Korreferenten: Prof. Dr. Vincent Heuveline, Dr. Stefanie Speidel

Impressum

KIT Scientific Publishing

Karlsruher Institut für Technologie (KIT)
KIT Scientific Publishing
Straße am Forum 2
D-76131 Karlsruhe

KIT Scientific Publishing is a registered trademark of Karlsruhe Institute of Technology. Reprint using the book cover is not allowed.

www.ksp.kit.edu

Print on Demand 2015

ISBN 978-3-7315-0373-6
DOI 10.5445/KSP/1000046886

Real-time Biomechanical Modeling for Intraoperative Soft Tissue Registration

zur Erlangung des akademischen Grades eines

Doktors der Ingenieurswissenschaften

der Fakultät für Informatik
des Karlsruher Instituts für Technologie (KIT)

genehmigte

Dissertation

von

Stefan Suwelack

aus Aachen

Tag der mündlichen Prüfung:	01.07.2014
Erster Gutachter:	Prof. Dr. Rüdiger Dillmann
Zweiter Gutachter:	Prof. Dr. Vincent Heuveline
Dritter Gutachter:	Dr. Stefanie Speidel

Abstract

Computer assisted surgery (CAS) systems intraoperatively support the surgeon by providing information on the location of hidden risk (e.g. vessels, nerves) and target structures (e.g. tumors) during surgery. In this way CAS techniques have been a major driving force for improving patient outcomes for many applications such as orthopedic surgery and neurosurgery. However, CAS is currently not used in the daily clinical routine for laparoscopic interventions. The main reason for this discrepancy are soft tissue deformations that make intraoperative registration (and thus intraoperative navigation) difficult. In this work, a novel, biomechanics based approach for real-time soft tissue registration from sparse intraoperative sensor data such as stereo endoscopic images was developed.

At the core of the method lies an accurate, yet real-time capable finite element (FE) model of the liver. For this purpose, a novel GPU based multigrid finite element solver is presented. The solver is based on a novel mapping scheme that allows to transfer displacements and forces between unstructured, non-conforming, higher order meshes. In order to achieve high efficiency on parallel hardware, a sparse approximate inverse approach is used for preconditioning and smoothing. By pre-computing and subsequently adapting this operator to the current deformation each time step, the approach becomes real-time capable.

In order to match the preoperative organ model to an intraoperative partial surface, the novel Physics based Shape Matching (PBSM) scheme is presented. This approach treats the non-rigid surface registration as an electrostatic-elastic problem, where an elastic body that is electrically charged (preoperative model) slides into an oppositely charged rigid shape (intraoperative surface). In contrast to previous attempts at biomechanically based registration, this novel physics based interpretation allows casting the shape matching problem into a single variational formulation. It is also the first method that employs a non-linear, yet real-time capable biomechanical model of the liver for registration purposes. In a large validation study based on numerical and phantom data, it was shown that the novel method outperforms state-of-the-art algorithms.

Further contributions of this work include methods for simulating tissue cutting during the intervention as well as new validation tools for CAS systems.

To my wife Eva-Maria

Acknowledgments

During my time as a research assistant at the Institute for Anthropomatics and Robotics I was very fortunate to meet many great individuals. They not only guaranteed that I had a great time during my PhD work, but also helped to shape this thesis by sharing ideas, opinions, criticism and scientific advise. Consequently, I am very thankful to many people for their support.

In particular I thank my thesis advisor Prof. Rüdiger Dillmann for giving me the opportunity to pursue a PhD. In addition to his scientific advise, I am very thankful to him for creating an inspiring work and research environment. Furthermore I greatly cherish his trust to give me the opportunity to teach during my PhD. I would like to express my sincere gratitude to Prof. Vincent Heuveline not only for agreeing to be the second reviewer for my thesis, but also for for the joint supervision of multiple student theses and his valuable advice in the realm of numerical methods. Furthermore, I thank Prof. Carsten Dachsbacher, Prof. Wolfgang Karl, Prof. Tanja Schultz and Prof. Bernhard Beckert for joining the examination board.

I would like to give very special thanks to Stefanie Speidel: First of all for excellent scientific guidance and for the thoughtful lead of the computer assisted surgery group. Also, for helping me to settle in into Karlsruhe, for lots of good restaurant recommendations and for plenty of baby-related support. I thank Michael Delles for making the overtime shifts in my first year enjoyable, for taking everything with a sense of humor and for being an expert in all dissertation related formalia. My thanks go to Sebastian Röhl not only for being a great roommate at the institute and during many retreats or conference trips, but also for our joint work at the MediAssist system. In this context, I would like to thank Gunther Sudra for starting MediAssist and Sebastian Bodenstedt, the godfather of MediAssist, for his enthusiasm, commitment and expertise during the system development. I thank Yoo-Jin Azad for many great talks about everything and Darko Katic for two fun MICCAI conferences and the latest guidelines on nutrition. I also thank Roland Unterhinninghofen for the opportunity to create the MedSim 2 lecture together.

Furthermore, I express my thanks to all members of the HIS/H2T institutes for helping to create such a great research environment. In particular, I thank Tamim Asfour for scientific advise. My thanks also

go to Marcus Strand, David Gonzalez and team captain Martin Do for all after-hours basketball activities (3rd place KABA cup!). I express my gratitude to Martin Lösch and Michael Neaga for the quick and efficient help for all server problems. Finally, I'm deeply indebted to our office team of Christine Brand, Diana Becker and Isabelle Wappler for their great patience and fantastic support.
This thesis could not have been completed without the commitment and expertise of the minimally invasive surgery group at the University Hospital Heidelberg. My thanks thus go to Martin Wagner, Hannes Kenngott, Anna-Laura Wekerle, Josephine Wünscher and Beat Müller for all the valuable advice and the joint work on the phantom experiments.
Furthermore, I thank Christian Sander, Manuel Serf and Julian Schill for their work on the SIMIO simulator. My thanks go to Dimitar Lukarski for the help on GPU solvers and to Markus Stoll for his great contributions to the MSML project.
During my time as a research assistant I had the privilege to mentor many great students. I thank all of them for their hard work, great questions and invaluable contributions to this thesis. In particular, I thank Tino Milschewski for his work on PBSM, Barbara Pfau and Maike Huber for their work on DG-FEM, Nicolai Schoch and Christoph Paulus for their work on X-FEM, Mario Laugisch and Philipp Stevermann for their work on GPU-based solvers as well as Hugo Talbot for his contributions to liver modeling (and a fun MMVR). I also thank Daniel Reichard for the image stitching component of MediAssist and Alexander Weigl for shaping MSML into a great software package.
I express my deepest thanks to all my friends and my family for their support. In particular, I thank my parents Waltraud and Prosper for all their encouragement and for sparking my interest in science. Finally, I thank my wife Eva-Maria for her infinite patience and for making everything special.

Karlsruhe, February 2015 Stefan Suwelack

Contents

The skill of writing is to create a context in which other people can think.
— Edwin Schlossberg

1. Introduction

Over the last decade computer assisted surgery (CAS) has become an invaluable tool in clinical practice. CAS (sometimes also called image guided surgery or computer assisted intervention) refers to using computer-based methods during intervention planning and execution. The main purpose of such systems is to intraoperatively support the surgeon by providing information on the location of hidden risk (e.g. vessels, nerves) and target structures (e.g. tumors) during surgery. In a similar fashion as navigation systems in a car help drivers to reach their destination in a fast and secure way, a CAS system guides a surgeon during the intervention. Here, preoperative planning data based on 3D tomographic images are used as a map of the patient. In analogy to the satellite position sensor used in a car navigation system, sensor data such as intraoperative imaging or tracking information is used to identify the hidden structures of interest within the surgical site. This allows the surgeon to remove tumors in an oncologically adequate manner while simultaneously preserving the surrounding healthy tissue. CAS technologies are especially beneficial in the context of minimally invasive surgery (MIS) as these procedures pose additional challenges to the surgeon such as a small surgical field, difficult hand-eye coordination and loss of 3D vision. In this context, CAS does not only help to reduce patient trauma and recovery time, but also facilitates the development of new operating techniques.

CAS methods are well established in the realm of neurosurgery and orthopedic surgery and have improved patient outcome [GWL99] [YC06]. However, such techniques are not currently used in clinical daily routine for most minimally invasive procedures in the abdominal cavity (so called laparoscopic interventions). In this context, intraoperative guidance

based on preoperative planning data remains a challenging problem. The main reason for this are soft tissue deformations caused by respiratory movement, heartbeat, pneumoperitoneum or surgical instruments. Due to these deformations the initial planning data significantly differs from the intraoperative patient anatomy. In order to accurately register the planning data to the patient (and thus provide a meaningful guidance), the soft tissue deformations have to be compensated in real-time.
For minimally invasive interventions, the available intraoperative data that can be used for registration purposes is usually very limited. In standard laparoscopy the endoscopic video image is the only available data source. With the advent of 3D monitors and robotic surgery systems, stereo endoscopes have been introduced into clinical practice. These systems allow reconstructing a 3D surface model of the surgical site [RBK+12]. However, they only provide information about the organ surfaces and not about internal motions (where the risk and target structures are located). Additional volumetric imaging modalities usually generate a higher overhead in terms of time and overall costs. Laparoscopic ultrasound (US) probes provide a cheap, but real-time capable image source [LVR+12]. However, not only is the resolution limited, but the probe only provides information in a particular image slice. More accurate imaging such as intraoperative C-arms do produce high resolution data, but require especially equipped operating rooms and special protocols due to radiation exposure [FMHN08]. In summary, especially these intraoperative sensors that integrate well into the surgical workflow do not provide enough resolution on the soft tissue deformations in time and/or space in order to provide meaningful guidance for many interventions. That's why the problem is also referred to as soft tissue registration based on sparse data.
In this thesis a new approach is developed that seeks to track soft tissue movements from sparse intraoperative sensor data by using a-priori information about the tissue's mechanical properties. At the heart of the approach is a real-time capable biomechanical model based on the finite element (FE) method. Different approaches are developed to recover the displacements of risk and target structures in real-time from stereo endoscopic image data. Furthermore, it is shown how the biomechanical model can be adapted during the intervention and a set of new methods for evaluating soft tissue registration algorithms is presented. The approach is applied to laparoscopic partial liver resection for evalua-

tion purposes. However, it is important to point out that variations of the method can be applied to many different laparoscopic soft tissue interventions.

1.1. Research questions

The primary objective of this work was to investigate if biomechanically based soft tissue registration is a viable approach for real-time intraoperative image guidance based on sparse sensor data. This general research goal can be broken down into the following different parts:

- **How does the complexity of the elasticity model influence the registration accuracy?**
  Many different biomechanical models have been proposed for different organs in the literature. They all differ in terms of complexity and parameterization. Especially with respect to real-time requirements, the question arises how complex (and thus computationally demanding) the model has to be in order to achieve a sufficient registration accuracy. In particular, it has to be investigated if a linear elasticity model is sufficient or if a non-linear model has to be used. Furthermore, it should be estimated if patient-specific parameter variations have a huge impact on the accuracy.

- **Can the model be solved numerically in real-time on operation room compatible hardware?**
  The elasticity based biomechanical model is discretized and solved numerically using the FE method. Here, it has to be determined which resolution is required in order to obtain sufficient accuracy. Furthermore, new methods have to be developed in order to make the computation more efficient. This in particular applies to the selection of suitable element technology. Also, the real-time model is much coarser than large-scale models typically used in engineering applications. It thus becomes feasible to use novel memory heavy pre-computations to speed up the computations. Special care has to be taken to design a suitable linear solver, as this is the most expensive part of the computation. Finally, it is interesting to investigate how the numerical performance can benefit from

massively parallel hardware (general purpose graphics processing units, GPGPU).

- **How can the information obtained from sensor data be accurately and efficiently imposed on the model?**
  The information obtained from intraoperative sensor data (e.g. displacements of organ surfaces) is imposed on the biomechanical model in terms of displacement boundary conditions and constraints. It is crucial for the registration accuracy that this is done in an accurate way. In particular, the following points are of interest: As points with known displacement do not necessarily coincide with the node positions of the coarse FE mesh, an efficient way has to be found to transfer these displacements. Also, the intraoperative sensor data can contain a significant amount of noise. Here, it is interesting to investigate how the biomechanical model can be used for regularization when the constraints are imposed in a soft way (e.g. through Robin boundary conditions). Finally, in a typical setting the boundary conditions are not completely known (e.g. the hidden side of the organs). Here, the question arises if it is viable to approximate these boundaries with simple models (e.g. zero displacement or zero traction).

- **How can the biomechanical model be updated in an efficient way during the intervention?**
  During many interventions the surgical scene changes significantly. This is in particular true if tissue is resected. In this case the changes to the organs have to be reflected in the biomechanical model in order to continuously provide a meaningful guidance. In the context of FE discretizations this means that the mesh has to be changed. Real-time re-meshing along arbitrary geometries (i.e. cut lines) is very challenging. In particular, the simulation can become unstable if ill-shaped elements (so-called sliver elements) are created. In this work, alternative methods are investigated that can embed discontinuities and geometry boundaries into existing grids without re-meshing. Instead, affected elements are enriched with more complex, discontinuous shape functions.

- **What are suitable validation protocols and tools for non-rigid soft tissue registration from sparse sensor data?**
  The validation of accuracy is a very important step towards a thorough evaluation for computer assisted surgery systems. In soft tissue interventions it is very complicated and sometimes even impossible to obtain reliable *in vivo* ground truth data. For this reason numerical simulations, organ phantoms and animal experiments are used as a means for validating the accuracy of CAS systems. A goal of this work is to develop a suitable validation strategy for the development of non-linear registration algorithms. In particular, tools for *in silico* and phantom based validation are investigated.

1.2. Contributions

Starting from the aforementioned research questions, a set of novel approaches, methods and algorithms has been developed. These include an efficient FE scheme based on quadratic tetrahedra and a fast GPU-based linear solver. Also, a novel physics-based shape matching approach and advanced techniques for cutting simulations resulted from this work. These algorithms and components are brought together into a novel prototype for biomechanically based real-time soft tissue registration. The most important contributions of this work on the algorithm and system level are:

Algorithms

- **Accurate surface embedding for higher order FE meshes:** For real-time deformable model simulation, high-resolution visualizations meshes have to be mapped to a low-resolution computational grid. In this work, a novel mapping scheme was introduced that generates smooth surface deformations and preserves local shape even for low-resolution computational meshes. It can be used to establish high quality mapping between higher order FE meshes for visualization purposes or to build multigrid hierarchies [SLH+13].

- **Fast GPU based solving scheme:** A novel multigrid scheme for solving quadratic FE-models on the GPU was developed. In order to achieve high efficiency on parallel hardware, a sparse approximate inverse approach is used for preconditioning and smoothing. In order to make this operator real-time capable, it is pre-computed and subsequently adapted to the current deformation each time step (*rotation warping*). The approach is the first to use a GPU-based multigrid scheme for solving real-time elasticity problems on higher-order unstructured grids.

- **Physics-based shape matching:** The novel physics-based shape matching (PBSM) approach can be used to robustly register intraoperatively acquired surface meshes (e.g. from stereo endoscopic, time-of-flight or ultrasound sensors) to preoperative planning data. The key idea of the method is to describe the non-rigid registration process as an electrostatic-elastic problem, where an elastic body (preoperative model) that is electrically charged slides into an oppositely charged rigid shape (intraoperative surface). As the technique is based on a preoperative volumetric FE model, it naturally recovers the position of volumetric structures (e.g. tumors, vessels) [SRB+14].

- **FE methods for flexible discontinuity and geometry embedding:** The adaptation of finite element meshes to geometry changes during the simulation (e.g. cracks, cuts) is challenging. In this thesis approaches based on the extended FEM (X-FEM) and the discontinuous Galerkin FEM (DG-FEM) are explored that solve this problem without re-meshing. In particular, a dynamic co-rotated X-FEM formulation for arbitrary cuts and an efficient coupling of enriched elements with the DG-FEM technique is presented. The methods can open up new approaches for embedding geometry into non-conforming meshes [PSS+14] [SSDH13].

Systems

- **Real-time biomechanical model for liver registration:** Starting from the available elasticity based liver models from the literature, several simulation studies were run to identify a suitable model for real-time registration [STR+11]. It was found that a co-rotational model based on quadratic tetrahedral elements offers the necessary performance while maintaining sufficient accuracy [SRD+11].

- **First prototype system for stable real-time FE based soft tissue registration in the context of laparoscopic liver resection:**The system combines stereo endoscopic and tracking data to derive constraints for a real-time biomechanical model. The system supports shape matching from pure geometric data for initial registration as well as texture based tracking for continuous real-time guidance. It was implemented as an extension to the MediAssist framework [SSRD10] [SKW+12] [SRB+14].

- **New set of validation tools for CAS:** Mechanically realistic silicon soft tissue phantoms were developed using parameter optimization approaches on FE models. These organ phantoms can be included in larger torso models to allow obtaining a reliable ground truth data for soft tissue registration scenarios. Furthermore, the results of this thesis contributed to a novel *in silico* evaluation tool for CAS. The developed validation workflows and tools initiated the launch of the open data validation platform www.open-cas.org [SRB+13].

- **The Medical Simulation Markup Language (MSML):** The MSML not only offers a generalized and flexible description for biomechanical simulation, but also for the workflow how the biomechanical model is constructed from tomographic data. In this way, the MSML can act as a middleware between all tools used in the modeling pipeline and thus greatly facilitates the prototyping of medical simulation workflows for clinical and research purposes [SSS+14].

1.3. Outline

The aim of this thesis is to detail and discuss the developed methods that have been outlined in the previous section. Due to the lack of established textbooks in the realm of both soft tissue simulation and real-time finite element methods, this text is self-contained. Thus, all major results of this thesis can be understood without the need of consulting further literature. In order to strike a balance between readability and mathematical rigor, further literature will be referenced where appropriate. The necessary fundamentals (e.g. elasticity theory, finite element methods, solver technology) are not introduced in separate chapters, but rather presented along the way where necessary to understand research results. Naturally, the first chapters will contain significant amounts of these fundamentals, while subsequent chapters focus purely on research results. The following chapters of this thesis are organized as follows:

- **Chapter 2** outlines the concept of biomechanically based soft tissue registration. For this purpose, some details on the medical example application (i.e. minimally invasive partial liver resection) are given. Furthermore, the specific components and techniques that have to be developed in order to realize this approach are discussed.

- Systems that use similar approaches are presented in **chapter 3**. Furthermore, the state of the art is discussed for all areas that are affected by the research that has been conducted in this thesis.

- A concise introduction to elasticity and soft tissue simulation is given in **chapter 4**. These fundamentals facilitate the numerical analysis of suitable biomechanical liver models.

- **Chapter 5** is dedicated to an in-depth introduction to the numerical solution of elasticity problems using finite element methods. Also, the efficient quadratic co-rotated tetrahedral FE formulation is presented.

- **Chapter 6** focusses on the presentation of a novel GPU based FE solver. The necessary fundamentals in solver technology (e.g. preconditioning, subspace and multigrid methods) are briefly introduced. Then the components of the new solver such as an efficient mapping scheme as well as highly parallel preconditioners and smoothers are detailed.

- A first prototype for stable real-time FE based soft tissue registration in the context of laparoscopic liver resection is presented in **chapter 7**. This includes the mathematical derivation of the novel physics-based shape matching scheme as well as a thorough validation of the system.

- The developed methods for simulating surgical cuts are discussed in **Chapter 8**. Based on an introduction to the X-FEM and the DG-FEM it is shown how cuts can be modeled without re-meshing. In particular a dynamic co-rotated X-FEM formulation for arbitrary cuts and an efficient coupling of enriched elements with the DG-FEM technique is presented.
- **Chapter 9** is dedicated to the most important tools that have been developed in the course of this research work and that are likely to have an impact on the future development of soft tissue simulation and registration techniques. These include validation techniques based on mechanically realistic soft phantoms and *in silico* evaluation tools, the web platform open-cas.org as well as the Medical Simulation Markup Language (MSML).
- A brief discussion of the presented research results along with some remarks about promising directions of future research that is sparked by the results of this thesis is presented in **chapter 10**.

Every great and deep difficulty bears in itself its own solution. It forces us to change our thinking in order to find it.
— Niels Bohr

2. An elasticity based approach to soft tissue registration

In this chapter, a novel approach for biomechanical model based soft tissue registration is outlined. In order to understand the special challenges that are associated with CAS systems for laparoscopic surgery, the first section will provide some background on laparoscopic partial liver resection. This intervention will serve as the showcase application throughout this thesis. In addition, the available intraoperative sensor data sources are described. We then outline a basic scheme for the initial registration of preoperative planning data with the patient in the OR and show how progressive real-time registration can be performed based on the initial alignment. The chapter concludes with an overview on the components that are necessary in order to implement the approach.

2.1. Laparoscopic partial liver resection

2.1.1. Laparoscopic interventions

In contrast to conventional open interventions, laparoscopic surgery is performed using long instruments that are inserted into the abdominal cavity through small skin incisions (Fig. 2.1). In the context of many interventions such as partial liver resection this approach has many benefits for the patient. It leads to faster recovery and significantly reduces complications and post-operative pain [RRA12]. However, due to reduced mobility as well as difficult depth perception and hand-eye coordination, minimally invasive interventions are especially challenging for surgeons [KDE$^+$12]. The fundamentally different operation technique and body posture require a significant training effort even for surgeons who are experienced in conventional techniques. For this reason, complex MIS interventions can greatly benefit from computer based assistance systems. By supporting the surgeon during the intervention (e.g. through the intraoperative visualization of preoperative planning data), the strain on the surgeon can be reduced. This helps to increase the accuracy as well as the quality of the intervention and the patient's safety [SBvDS12].

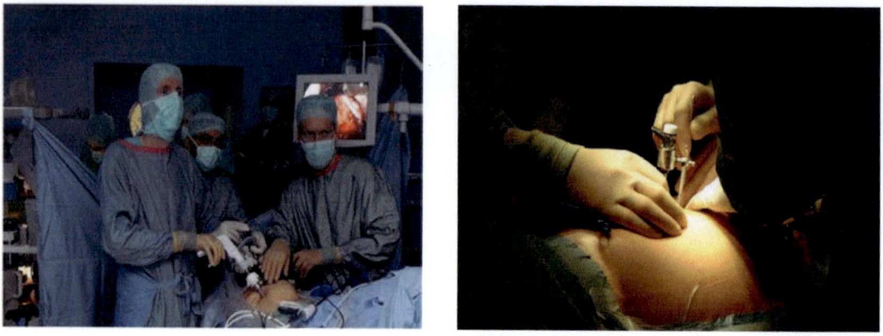

Figure 2.1.: In order to perform laparoscopic surgery (left) the abdomen has to be inflated with carbon dioxide (right) [©Heidelberg University Hospital].

The novel registration methods developed in this thesis are exemplarily evaluated in the context of laparoscopic partial liver resection. The purpose of this minimally invasive intervention is the removal of liver tumors. In a recent study on 2466 patients, Rao et al. compared laparoscopic partial liver section to the conventional open approach. They showed that the laparoscopic technique leads to a reduced mortality rate, less positive resection margins of malign operations as well as a reduced amount of blood transfusions [RRA12]. Despite these results, the conventional open surgery is the standard procedure in many clinical centers. Among the reasons for the slow adoption of the MIS technique are the more difficult operating technique, increased training requirements and a more difficult tumor localization due to the heavily reduced tactile sense [GAA$^+$12]. Furthermore, the access to central liver metastases is often difficult in the laparoscopic setting. Consequently, Nguyen et al. found that 65% of all published literature on laparoscopic liver resection deal with special cases that are easier to perform (45% are atypical wedge resection and 20% are left lateral segment resections) [NGG09]. In this context, a CAS system could help to make central liver metastases treatable in a minimally invasive way.

2.1.2. Liver anatomy

The liver is located in the upper abdomen right below the diaphragm and is protected by the lower rib cage. It is the largest internal organ and weighs about 1.2-1.4kg in healthy adult females and about 1.4-1.8kg in adult males [Lip11]. Surrounded by the collagenous Glisson capsule, the liver is an extremely vascular organ. Oxygen rich blood is supplied through the Hepatic artery, while nutrient rich blood from the gastrointestinal tract flows into the liver through the portal vein. The blood returns to the heart through the left, middle and right hepatic vein which coalesce into the vena cava. Due to the high amount of blood flow, the liver is especially susceptible to metastatic tumors [Per07]. It was discovered by C. Couinaud that the liver can be divided into eight functionally independent segments [BCG+00]. During partial resection, it is very important to keep enough segments alive in order to preserve the functionality of the liver. That is why cut lines have to be placed along the edges of the Couinaud segments. This requires very accurate planning and execution, making liver surgery an excellent application for CAS methods.

2.1.3. Hepatic motion

During free breathing, the liver is subjected to significant motion. In a meta study, Clifford et al. found that the respiratory motion strongly varies between individuals in terms of magnitude and direction [CBLC02]. The most significant motion occurs in the cranio-caudal direction with magnitudes ranging from 10 mm to 26 mm. It should be pointed out that the liver does not undergo a pure whole organ translation, but is subjected to considerable non-rigid deformation. Thus, peak displacements inside the liver can reach up to 34 mm and registration errors up to 15 mm occur, if a pure rigid registration is performed [RMOZ04]. In addition to respiration induced motion, cardiovascular

activity changes the position of the liver. However, with a magnitude of less than 1 mm this effect is comparably small [KMAB04].
The hepatic motion during laparoscopic surgery is significantly different. First of all, the abdomen is insufflated with carbon dioxide in order to create enough operating space in preparation of laparoscopic interventions. This so called pneumoperitoneum severely changes the intraoperative position of the liver in comparison with the preoperative position during CT imaging [FMHN08]. Thus, an initial non-rigid alignment is needed at the beginning of the intervention in order to compensate this effect. Furthermore, the liver is often moved from its original location using laparoscopic instruments or retractors during surgery. This is the primary source of liver motion during the intervention and leads to large deformations. Finally, the respiratory motion is strongly attenuated due to the pneumoperitoneum.

2.2. Available intraoperative sensor data

By definition, laparoscopic surgery is not possible without an endoscope. In clinical routine, monoscopic endoscopes are typically used. However, starting with the adoption of the daVinci telemanipulation system, stereo endoscopes became widely available (see Fig. 2.2) [MMD+04]. These endoscopes do not only provide the surgeon with a three dimensional view on the surgical site (thus alleviating a major drawback of MIS), but they also enable the development of powerful computer vision algorithms. Based on the stereo images, it is possible to perform instrument and soft tissue tracking [MY12]. Furthermore, a complete 3D reconstructions of the surgical site can be obtained [RBS+12]. With the advent of affordable and easy-to-use 3D monitors, adoption of stereo endoscopic technology in daily clinical routine is increasing [SBKK12]. New developments such as chip-on-the-tip and LED lighting help to continuously increase the image quality and resolution. Thus, it is to be expected that stereo endoscopes will remain the primary sensor source for CAS in the laparoscopic context in the near future. However, alternative sensors such as time-of-flight endoscopes or structured light approaches exist, but are not used in clinical practice yet [MHMB+13].
Accurate tracking of the patient and important surgery devices such as needles, instruments or endoscopes is very important for every CAS

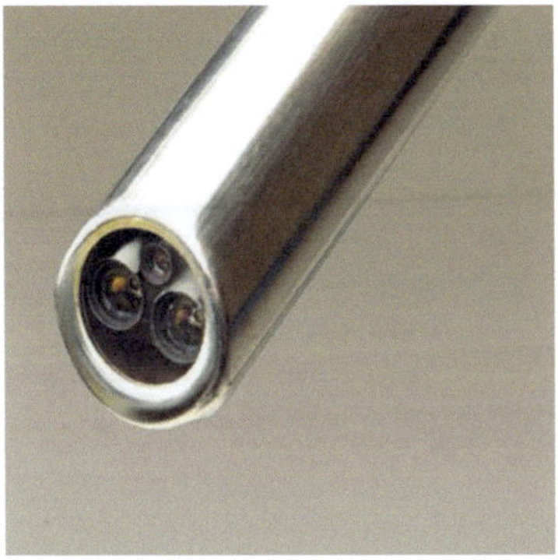
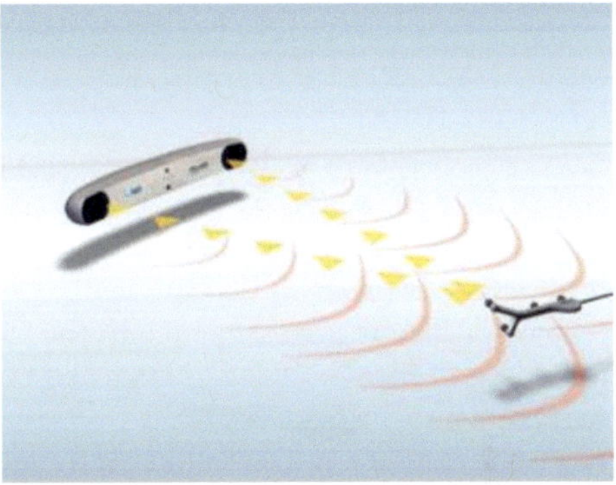

Figure 2.2.: Stereo endoscope from the daVinci telemanipulation system (left) [©Intuitive Surgical, Inc.] and optical tracking system NDI Polaris Aurora (right) [©Northern Digital, Inc.].

system. A common approach is to use a stereo camera system and an infrared light source to track small marker balls that can be attached to surgical devices. These optical tracking systems such as the NDI Polaris (see Fig. 2.2) achieve sub-millimeter accuracy and are used in many commercial CAS systems (e.g. BrainLab [GWL99] for neurosurgery). A major drawback of the optical tracking is the line of sight requirement. This condition is often difficult to fulfill in the OR setting. That's why electromagnetic tracking systems are used for many interventions. However, they do not achieve the same accuracy as optical trackers and can suffer from noise and distortion if metallic or electrical devices are within the tracking range. Other promising tracking technology that hasn't been used in the OR yet are radio frequency identification (RFID) based chips and small, wireless accelerometers.
In terms of volumetric imaging modalities, 2D laparoscopic ultrasound (US) is often used for intraoperative guidance [LVR+12]. It is cheap, provides real-time information and can be integrated into the surgical workflow reasonably well. Information from 2D ultrasound probes can be combined into 3D images for intraoperative soft tissue registration and guidance [NHS+07]. However, 2D ultrasound has several drawbacks. Not only is the field of view limited, but the trocar placement in laparoscopic surgery can make it difficult to obtain a complete overview

of the organ [LVR+12]. Furthermore, the image quality of US is much lower if compared to CT and MRI due to a low signal-to-noise ratio and reflection artifacts.
A very accurate way to obtain volumetric images is to use special OR-compatible X-ray devices called C-arms. These systems are particularly well suited in order to obtain an initial registration of planning data [FMHN08] [KWG+13b]. However, this technology is still relatively expensive, it needs a lot of space in the OR and can only be used a limited number of times in order to keep the radiation exposure low for patients, surgeons and nurses.
The goal of this work is to research new model based techniques for soft tissue registration based on limited intraoperative sensor data. These methods ultimately aim at providing guidance without the invasive, expensive and/or time consuming use of additional complex intraoperative imaging modalities. That is why throughout this thesis, all approaches will be based on only stereo endoscopic and tracking data. However, we point out that the developed techniques can easily be extended to include other intraoperative data such as US.

2.3. Surface based registration

2.3.1. Initial registration

In this section we sketch a biomechanically based approach to register planning data to the patient at the beginning of the intervention. This technique relies on a **biomechanical model** of the liver which is built from segmented CT or MRI data. During the intervention, the method uses an **intraoperative 3D surface model** of the liver which is obtained from the **sensor data** using suitable 3D reconstruction, image stitching and texture based segmentation techniques. The goal is to align the biomechanical model with the intraoperative surface. In other words, the **boundary conditions** (i.e. forces or displacements on the surface of the model) have to be determined in such a way, that the deformed model matches the intraoperative surface as best as possible (see Fig. 2.3).
In this work we propose the **physics-based shape matching** (PBSM) approach to establish the shape correspondence between preoperative and intraoperative data and to determine the appropriate boundary condi-

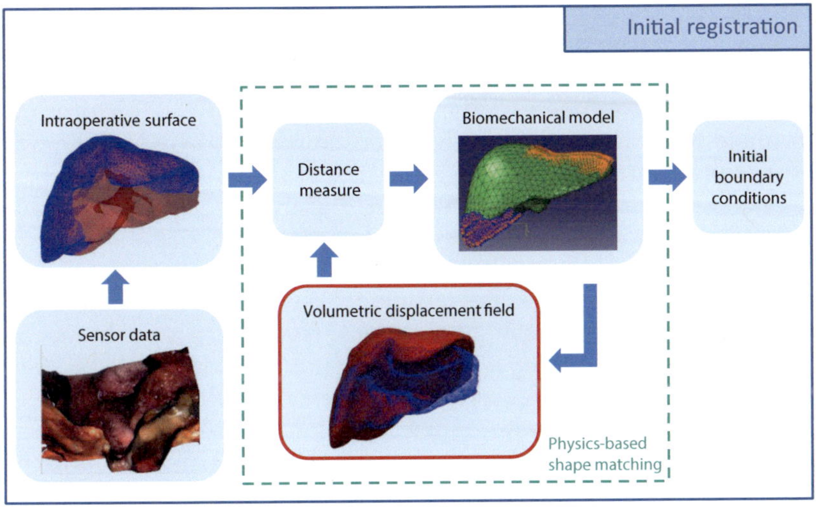

Figure 2.3.: Scheme for initial alignment of preoperative planning data based on tomographic imaging with intraoperative endoscopic images.

tions. More specifically, the non-rigid registration process is regarded as an electrostatic-elastic problem, where an elastic body (preoperative model) that is electrically charged slides into an oppositely charged rigid shape (intraoperative surface). In other words, a suitable **distance measure** (Fig. 2.3) drives the deformation while the biomechanical model acts as a regularization term. The scheme does recover the full **volumetric displacement field** and does not need any known correspondences (i.e. landmarks). However, any landmark based approach can be used to enhance the accuracy of PBSM by connecting the known landmarks with stiff springs.

In the intraoperative setting, organ surfaces are only partially visible. Naturally, the question arises how the boundary condition on the hidden surface should be modeled. A straight forward approach is to use a-priori information about the movement of organ surfaces. In accordance with results from the literature ([CMG+07], [HDP+13]), we fix areas with negligible motion during the registration. In order to further enhance the

registration accuracy, the PBMS approach can be used in an optimization scheme to estimate the unknown boundary conditions. For this purpose, different characteristic surface regions should be defined (e.g. surface connected to diaphragm). Then the unknown surface forces can be assumed to be constant on each surface in order to avoid an ill-posed inverse problem.
As explained in the previous section, the liver is still affected from respiratory motion in the laparoscopic setting. As this movement is comparatively small, it will be neglected in the evaluations that are presented in this thesis. As the respiratory movement is periodic, the extension from the static setting to dynamic boundaries is straight forward. Using the signal from the medical ventilator, a dynamic model of the intraoperative liver surface can be spatio-temporally registered with the preoperative data. This registration results in dynamic (moving) initial boundary conditions.

2.3.2. Landmark based progressive real-time registration

Having established an initial correspondence between intraoperative and preoperative data (and thus having computed the initial **boundary conditions**), texture based **soft tissue tracking** can be used to determine the displacement on the liver surface (Fig. 2.4). Although it is possible to directly impose the observed displacements as Dirichlet (pure displacement boundary conditions), it is usually a better idea to impose them in a weaker way as Robin boundary conditions. Physically, this can be interpreted as connecting the landmarks through springs with the organ's surface.

2.4. A system for biomechanically based soft tissue registration

In this section, we discuss the basic components that have to be developed in order to design a system that implements the presented registration approach. The discussion in particular links these components to the corresponding chapters in this thesis and thus serves as a natural extension to the thesis outline given in section 1.3.

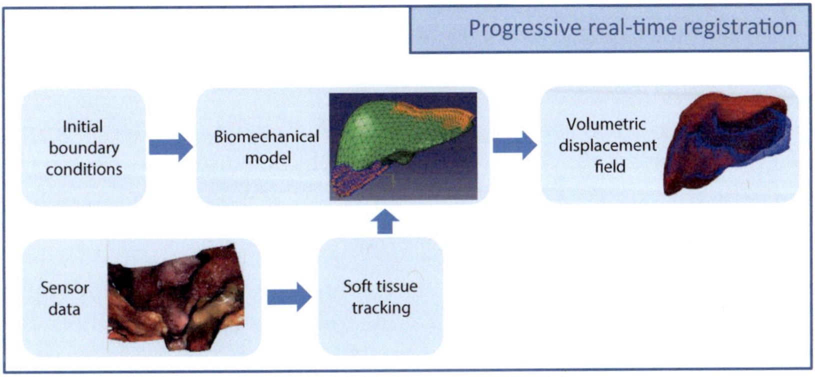

Figure 2.4.: Scheme for progressive real-time guidance using texture based feature tracking and biomechanical modeling.

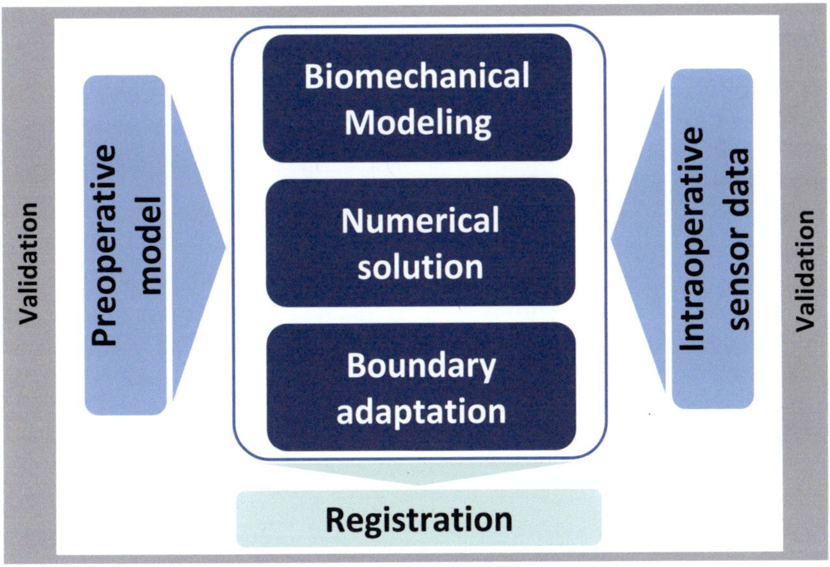

Figure 2.5.: Components of a system for biomechanically based soft tissue registration.

Fig. 2.5 shows the main system components. At the heart of the approach lies a real-time capable, **accurate biomechanical model**. The first step in the development is the identification of a suitable elasticity model which is extensively discussed in chapter 4. A critical challenge is the robust, **real-time numerical solution** of the identified model. In order to achieve that goal, efficient FE discretizations have to be employed (see chapter 5). Furthermore, new linear solvers have to be developed that are able to harness the computing power of massively parallel hardware (chapter 6). The most important component of the system is the actual **registration** of the **preoperative biomechanical model** with the **intraoperative sensor data**. This means computing the initial boundary conditions and subsequently adapting the boundary based on texture tracking. In the developed prototype system, this is achieved using the novel physics-based shape matching scheme (chapter 7). In practice, the construction of suitable biomechanical models from **preoperative tomographic data** is very time consuming. That is why new tools for simplifying this biomechanical modeling workflow can significantly speed up development and validation of biomechanically based approaches (chapter 9). Finally, the biomechanical model has to be adapted according to changes in the surgical scene. In addition to current force and displacement boundary conditions, this often means **adapting the boundary** of the geometry itself (e.g. due to cutting). Possible solutions to this problem are discussed in chapter 8.

In addition to CAS system design, its **accurate validation** is crucial for further development and clinical use. In this context it is particularly challenging to generate reliable and repeatable validation set-ups with known ground truth deformations. In this work, the validation is based on sophisticated phantoms (e.g. chapter 7). A detailed view on mechanically accurate soft tissue phantoms is given in chapter 9. In the same chapter we discuss the impact of open validation data and suitable platforms for data sharing and benchmarking.

If a man will begin with certainties, he shall end in doubts; but if he will be content to begin with doubts he shall end in certainties
— Francis Bacon

3. State of the art

In this chapter we discuss the state of the art for all research areas that are relevant to this work. Initially, possible medical applications in the realm of kidney, prostate, heart and liver surgery and their specific challenges are discussed. Along the way current CAS approaches for these interventions are presented with a strong emphasis on biomechanically based methods. As surface-to-surface registration (or shape matching) is an important component in the system, the relevant background for rigid and non-rigid surface matching is subsequently discussed. It has already been pointed out that the focus of this work is to develop suitable biomechanical models for the registration process. Thus, typical approaches to biomechanical modeling for abdominal organs will be discussed and an extensive review on current real-time FE modeling techniques is presented. Current methods for simulating surgical cuts are subsequently introduced. Finally, we take a look at validation techniques for CAS systems.

3.1. Computer assisted interventions

Computer based intraoperative image guidance helps surgeons to precisely visualize and target the surgical site by providing critical information during the intervention. Typically, this means to intraoperatively display preoperative planning data using suitable visualization techniques such as augmented reality [BFMR08]. Although this approach is well established in orthopedics and neurosurgery, it is still not widely used in the laparoscopic setting. Both Peters et al. [PC08] and Cleary et al. [CP10] identify the difficult compensation of soft tissue movements as a primary reason for this development.

3.1.1. Neurosurgery

In order to provide meaningful computer guidance during craniectomy, the arising nerve tissue movements (*brain shift*) have to be compensated [SSND01]. In this context, biomechanical models have first been applied to intraoperative registration. Warfield et al. presented an algorithm based on a linear elasticity model [CDT+05]. A stereo camera system is used to derive the displacement on the brain's surface and the finite element method is employed to solve the ensuing boundary problem. The group was able to demonstrate in a patient study that the registration error could be reduced from 7.4 mm to 1.8 mm if compared to a rigid registration technique [ACW+07]. Miller et al. have improved on this work by exploring more elaborate biomechanical models [Mil00]. In particular, they used a non-linear, patient-specific biomechanical model for brain shift compensation [WMKW07]. When compared to intraoperative MRI measurements, the registration showed a maximal error of 1 mm. The group also presented a very interesting comparison of different material models in order to estimate the influence of the model complexity on the registration result [HWM06]. The study shows that viscoelastic effects have only minimal impact on the solution. However, there is a big difference between a geometric non-linear (and thus rotation-invariant) model and a linear material model. Thus, it can be concluded that the typically used linear models limit the obtainable registration accuracy for the brain shift problem [WHM09].

3.1.2. Laparoscopic partial nephrectomy

For partial nephrectomy (partial resection of the kidney) only an initial registration is necessary as soft tissue movement during the intervention is minimal. In this context Nakamura et al. presented a manual registration approach in order to generate an augmented reality overlay in the endoscopic video [NNZ+10]. An improved method was developed by Pratt et al. [PMV+12]. Here, the surgeon picks a landmark in the preoperative mesh using ray intersection and then selects the same landmark in the video image. By using a stereo endoscope, the system can then derive the intraoperative 3D point and matches it to the preoperative data. The final rotational alignment is done manually using a special 3D input device. The work also includes a hardware platform for displaying augment reality visualization on the daVinci telemanipulation system. One possibility to automate the registration step is to use small navigation markers around the structure of interest. Intraoperatively, these markers are initially registered to the planning data using volumetric imaging. Baumhauer et al. presented such a system for computer assisted partial nephrectomy [BFMR08]. They use 4 navigation markers and a Siemens Arcadis C-arm device for intraoperative registration. The markers are subsequently tracked in endoscopic images in order to generate an overlay image in the endoscopic view. An *in silico* and *in vitro* evaluation of the results showed good tracking stability and reasonable accuracy of the approach. For a recent review on CAS methods in the context of partial nephrectomy we also refer to Hughes-Hallett et al. [HHMM+13].

3.1.3. Laparoscopic prostatectomy

The resection of tumors in the prostate (prostatectomy) is a common use case for robotic surgery. In 2012, around 80% of prostatectomies in the US were performed using robotic assistance [SHHM+13]. Typically, diagnosis and preoperative planning is done based on magnetic resonance (MR) imaging [HAT+12]. One possibility is to additionally use intraoperative MRI for guidance [PFtH+08]. However, this is not only very expensive, but the intraoperative MRI is of much lower quality than the preoperative images. Furthermore, image acquisition is slow and MR compatible operating equipment has to be used. In contrast, intraoperative 3D transrectal ultrasound (TRUS) is comparably cheap, easy to use and provides real-time data on the surgical site. In order to use MR based preoperative data in this context, it has to be registered to the TRUS image. In addition to manual registration [SKX+08] several automatic registration approaches have been proposed for this purpose. Alterovitz et al. proposed a FE based technique [AGP+06]. For this purpose they employ a 2D linear elastic FE model for each segmented MRI slice. The boundary conditions as well as material parameters are estimated by using a steepest descent optimization algorithm on top of the biomechanical model. Crouch et al. presented a method to register segmented prostate surfaces [CPC+07]. The approach makes use of medial shape models in order to get compute an initial guess of the boundary conditions. The accurate boundary conditions are then

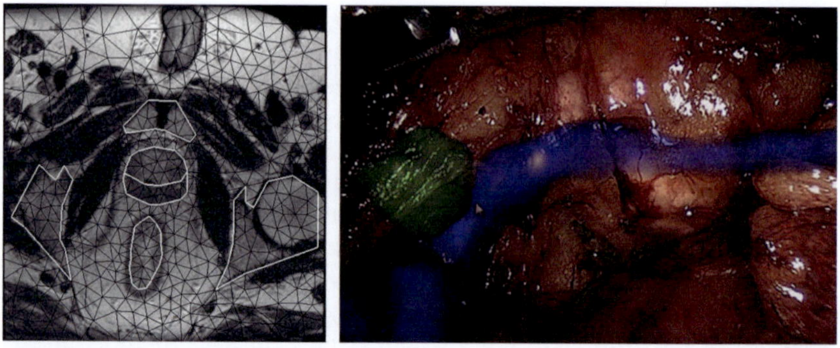

Figure 3.1.: FE based registration of MR slices for soft tissue registration in the context of prostatectomy (right) [AGP+06] and manual overlay of a tumor and a vessel during laparoscopic partial liver resection (right) [NSMM11].

estimated using a Nelder-Mead simplex search algorithm. More recently, Hu et al. used biomechanical modeling to learn a statistical shape model (SSM) that represents all possible deformations and used the SSM to derive a dense deformation field from the US sensor data.

3.1.4. MIS at the heart

For minimally invasive interventions at the heart, image guidance based on preoperative data is still in in development state. One possibility is to use US imaging of the heart (echocardiography) for guidance [KVPP10]. An interesting research area in this context seeks is the motion compensation of the beating heart's surface using robotic technology. The idea behind this methods is to track the movement of the heart's surface in video images [SY07]. In order to robustly estimate dense displacement fields on the heart, pseudo-physical models such as thin plate splines [RPL08] or finite element based biomechanical models can be employed [BPH11].

Pratt et al. presented a biomechanically based approach for real-time intraoperative soft tissue registration for MIS interventions at the heart [PSVSY10]. They use temporally resolved 4D-CT data in order to build a 3D model of the heart's movement. The forces on the heart's surface are then determined using a FE model. Instrument-induced displacements on the surface are obtained using feature tracking in stereo endoscopic images and the total deformation of the organ is finally computed by superimposing the tracked displacements with the previously computed forces. For this registration process, Pratt et al. use a non-linear biomechanical model which is solved using FE and explicit time integration. A big drawback of this method is the poor stability of the time integration technique. Thus, it is not possible to reliably simulate all deformations that typically arise during an intervention.

3.1.5. Conventional liver surgery

The group of Cash et al. has investigated biomechanical model based compensation of soft tissue movements during open liver interventions [CMS+05] [CMG+07]. They use a laser range scanner in order to obtain an intraoperative surface of the liver. This surface is then imposed on a linear elasticity FE model using so called *closest point* boundary conditions: Here, the intraoperative surface is first rigidly registered to the preoperative model. Subsequently, the position of each FE node on the *closest point* boundary is set to the displacement of the closest point in the intraoperative surface mesh. If only the displacement in normal direction is imposed, the boundary of the FE model is free to slide along the intraoperative surface. In this way an exact match can be computed through an iterative process. This approach was enhanced by Dumpuri et al. and Simpson et al. [DCDM10] [SDJM12] in two critical aspects. First, the initial rigid registration is performed using the weighted patch ICP (see previous section) in order to improve the stability and accuracy of the process. Furthermore, the correspondences between the intraoperative surface and the FE mesh are established by solving a Laplace equation on the surface of the undeformed FE grid. More recently, Rucker et al. showed an approach to estimate the boundary conditions on the unknown surface [RWC+13]. They describe the boundary conditions in terms of a bivariate polynomial form and use a Levenberg-Marquardt procedure to optimize its position. In the context of open liver surgery, the liver is usually de-mobilized. Thus it is only necessary to derive an initial match between preoperative and intraoperative data. That is why the presented algorithms are not aimed at progressive real-time motion compensation.

3.1.6. Laparoscopic partial liver resection

The design of CAS systems for laparoscopic interventions at the liver is especially difficult. Here, it is not only necessary to obtain an accurate initial registration, but it is also necessary to compensate ongoing tissue movements due to instruments and respiration in real-time. Nicolau et al. showed that manual overlays can be feasible if the field of view is very limited. However, they identify the automatic, progressive registration during the intervention as a central building block for a CAS system in the context of laparoscopic liver surgery [NSMM11]. The most common approach to intraoperative guidance for liver surgery is to use ultrasound as an additional intraoperative modality. Nakamoto et al. equipped a laparoscopic 2D US probe with a magnetic tracking marker [NHS+07]. With this setup, they were able to register the 2D slices spatially and temporally and obtain a 4D dataset of the liver. A similar approach was presented and evaluated by Sahin et al. [SBKS14]. Instead of registering preoperatively obtained tomographic data to the intraoperative image, they directly segment the tumor in the obtained US data. On big drawback of this approach is that it is not possible to generate an intraoperative visualization of important planning data such as cut paths or the position of important vessels. For more information on the use of laparoscopic ultrasound for abdominal soft tissue interventions we refer to the review paper by Lango et al. [LVR+12].
Intraoperative X-ray imaging by means of a C-arm system has also been proposed to initially align the intraoperative surgical site with preoperative data [FMHN08] [KWG+13b]. However, this approach does not only require complex intraoperative imaging, it also exposes patients, physicians and nurses to radiation. Furthermore, this technique does not allow for progressive real-time tracking of soft tissue deformations.
More recently Haouchine et al. presented a biomechanically based approach for real-time liver registration [HDP+13]. They use a stable co-rotational model in conjunction with implicit time integration. In this way, the model is sufficiently accurate and stable. They show that texture based tissue tracking can be used to maintain correspondences between preoperative and intraoperative models for short periods of time. However, not only is a necessary initial registration missing in these attempts, but the method is also very susceptible to modifications of the surgical scene (e.g. blood).

3.1.7. Radiation therapy

In the context of radiation therapy, soft tissue motion compensation is a highly relevant research area for treatment areas such as the lungs or abdominal organs. Here, we only mention these approaches that are methodically relevant to this work. A simple, yet efficient approach to compensate respiratory induced motion was introduced by Hostettler et al. [HNF+06] [HNS+08]. This technique uses an incompressibility assumption for the abdominal organs in order to derive a dense displacement field. Although only a simple phenomenological approach is used, the reported errors are less than 3 mm. A more elaborate approach is used by Brock et al. in order to register tomographic images in inspiration and expiration [BSD+05]. They use the commercial software Hypermorph in an iterative scheme in order to derive boundary conditions for a FE elasticity model.

3.2. Surface registration and shape matching

Many types of intraoperative sensor data such as stereo endoscopic, time-of-flight or laser range scanner data can be used to reconstruct 3D surface models of the surgical site [Sto12] [DCDM10] [RBS+12] [MHMB+13]. In this context non-rigid registration of two triangular meshes (sometimes referred to as *shape matching* or *shape correspondence*) has to be performed in order to provide image guidance. The shape matching is especially challenging in the intraoperative setting due to noisy sensor data, only partially visible surfaces, ambiguous shape descriptors and the requirement to keep the computation time low.

The registration problem can be tackled by directly searching for pairwise correspondence, by first computing an aligning transformation between the two shapes or by an iterative combination of these approaches (hybrid methods) [KZHCO10]. The iterative closes point (ICP) algorithm uses a simple, yet efficient hybrid scheme for rigid point cloud registration [YM92]: For each iteration, correspondence is established using the nearest-neighbor relationship. The best-fit transformation is subsequently derived by minimizing the distances of corresponding points in a least-squares sense. Although the ICP is guaranteed to converge, it often converges to a local minimum and not to the global best-fit solution.

Thus, a good starting pose is crucial for the algorithm's performance. Several improvements have been made to address this problem [RL01]. A good approach is to directly establish correspondence pairs (e.g. through graph matching [dSGF+12] or voting techniques [LF09]) in order to compute a good initial pose before running the ICP. As demonstrated in the weighted-patch ICP variant, it is also possible to include landmark-based techniques directly into the ICP formulation [CCD+08].
For non-rigid shape matching a dense set of corresponding feature points has to be found. Additionally, the global consistency of a non-rigid transformation is usually ensured by adding a regularization term to the minimization criterion [KZHCO10]. Different types of regularization (e.g. geodesic distance, transformation similarity) have been proposed in the literature [KZHCO10]. Although deformation based regularization measures have been investigated [CR03] [ZSCO+08] no attempt has been made thus far to use a biomechanical model for that purpose.
An interesting approach to point set registration was presented by Myronenko et al. [MS10]. They treat the registration process as a probability density estimation problem. The problem is solved by fitting Gaussian mixture model centroids (first point set) to the data (second point set) by maximizing the likelihood. This approach called *coherent point drift* algorithm was extended to include non-rigid matching by using a regularization term that ensures the smoothness of the deformation. For an extensive review of current rigid and non-rigid surface registration techniques we refer to Tam et al. [TCL+13].
In this thesis the novel physics based shape matching algorithm is proposed. We describe non-rigid surface registration as an electrostatic-elastic problem, where an elastic body that is electrically charged (preoperative model) slides into an oppositely charged rigid shape (intraoperative surface). The idea of using electric potentials to match objects has already been explored for rigid alignment [CSLY01] and in the context of shape recovery [JWR04].

3.3. Biomechanical modeling of abdominal organs

3.3.1. Elasticity based material models

Many different continuum mechanics based material models with vastly different complexity levels have been proposed for soft tissue. In contrast to the simple linear models that have been used in the previously presented registration approaches, accurate soft tissue simulation usually requires non-linear modeling [Fun93]. Models have been proposed for many organs and tissue types such as the liver [NMHB04] [RES10] [KS05] or the brain [MC97] [Mil00]. The dynamical behavior of soft tissue is typically modeled using viscoelastic approaches. The models are usually parameterized by subjecting organs to pre-defined forces and measuring the resulting deformation using volumetric imaging. In this context, some methods have been proposed for *in-vivo* analysis of the tissue. These approaches allow to determine a patient-specific parameterization during the intervention. Jordan et al. showed how a parameter identification technique on top of a finite element model can be used to parameterize a porcine liver model from 3D ultrasound data [JSZH09]. During the *in vitro* experiment the group used artificial perfusion in order to mimic *in vivo* conditions. A similar approach based on a stereo camera system instead of 3D US was presented by Lister et al. [LGD10].

3.3.2. Biomechanical workflow

Using elasticity theory, the continuum mechanics based models can be mathematically formulated as a boundary value problem. This is typically solved numerically using discretization techniques (e.g. the FE method) that require a volumetric computational grid to be generated. This workflow consists of several stages: Segmentation, surface meshing, mesh cleaning, volumetric meshing, definition of boundary conditions and material properties. Different software tools exist for each of these steps. There are many established open-source packages for segmentation [PHK04] [TSF+07] [WVW+05], mesh processing [CCC+08], volumetric meshing [FP09], biomechanical simulation [FDD+12] and post processing [HAL04]. Commercial CAE packages such as Materialise

Mimics and 3matics, ABAQUS and Ansys are also frequently used in biomechanics applications.
Some software packages combine segmentation, meshing, simulation and post-processing capabilities into a single application [MEAW12] [PHK04]. Furthermore, the Monitor Markup Language (MML) was integrated into the CamiTK framework in order to facilitate the comparison between different simulation backends and modeling approaches [FDKP12]. However, currently there is no modeling language that can represent the whole biomechanical modeling workflow. Furthermore, the presented systems are not easily expandable without in-depth knowledge of the respective framework.
Some simulation frameworks like SOFA use elaborate XML-based formats to model biomechanical simulations [FDD+12]. However, there is currently no standardized format for describing material properties, boundary conditions or simulation parameters. During the development of the medical simulation markup language (MSML) that is presented in this thesis, we looked at the following markup schemes: The Virtual Reality Modeling Language is an XML-based description for physical objects [CB97]. In the medical field, the Medical Reality Modeling Language can represent typical data arising in image-guided surgery [GNK+01]. The Surgical Simulation and Training Markup Language (SSTML) describes surgical workflows and organ models for surgery training [BTPE06]. In the context of biomechanical simulation, the Physical Model Language (PML) was designed to achieve a unified formulation of both FE and mass spring models [CP04]. It should be pointed out that, in contrast to MSML, none of the presented approaches allow for flexible extension (e.g. towards new material models) or compatibility checking.

3.4. Real-time finite element modeling

3.4.1. Model-order reduction techniques

One possibility to simulate non-linear, viscoelastic models in real-time is to rely on extensive pre-computations. This approach is taken by model-order-reduction techniques based on eigenvalue computations [BJ05] [NACC08] or statistical analysis [KRS09] [MKSN+12]. Clements et al. even propose to build an atlas for all deformations that can occur during an intervention and to compute the intraoperative solution through linear combinations of these pre-computed deformation patterns [CDC+07]. All these approaches have the big drawback of becoming invalid as soon as the model is substantially changed (e.g. due to surgical cutting) during the intervention. Furthermore, it is difficult to predict the soft tissue deformations caused by surgical instruments.

3.4.2. Explicit time integration

One method for directly solving the biomechanical model in real-time was presented by Miller et al. The group used a FE approach in the total Lagrange formulation in conjunction with low order elements and an explicit time integration scheme (*total Lagrangian explicit dynamics* - TLED) [MJLW07]. Joldes et al. presented a extension of the approach that significantly reduces the volume locking effect [JWM08]. Taylor et al. demonstrated the inherent parallel nature of the algorithm with an efficient implementation on graphics hardware (GPU) [TCO08] [TCC+08] [CP08].

3.4.3. Fully non-linear models with implicit time integration

The explicit time integration scheme is only stable, if the time step is sufficiently small. Depending on the boundary conditions, this stable time step can become extremely small, thus rendering the method very inefficient despite its small computation time per time step. In contrast, the time step can often be several orders of magnitudes larger if implicit time integration is used.
However, a discrete formulation of non-linear elastic models based on an implicit time integration technique requires a non-linear system solve during each time step. This typically means an iterative solve of linear systems (Newton-Raphson approach) and re-computing the stiffness matrix for every iteration. The multiplicative Jacobian energy decomposition (MJED) approach presented by Marchesseau et al. allows for a very fast computation of the stiffness matrix. However, the approach still needs several linear system solve per time step.

3.4.4. Corotated finite elements

Corotated finite elements offer a promising alternative to fully non-linear elasticity models [FH05]. The idea of this approach is to extract the rotational component of the deformation gradient and then use a linear material law. The resulting formulation is rotation-invariant, but only requires one linear system solve per time step. In the realm of computer graphics corotated FE have become an established method for physically and visually accurate interactive simulation of deformable models [HS04] [MG04]. It is well known that quadratic tetrahedra perform much better than linear tetrahedral elements in many engineering applications [CK92]. This is in particular true for the simulation of incompressible objects. However, despite the widespread use of FE based simulations in computer graphics, only three groups have investigated quadratic volumetric FE in the context of real-time deformable models [KMBG09][MTPS09][WKS+11]. They all concluded that higher order elements are superior to linear elements in terms of speed and accuracy.
The primary reason that prevents the use of higher order FE methods for real-time deformable model simulation is the much more difficult integration into the visualization pipeline. In addition to a more difficult grid generation, it is in particular challenging to accurately map high resolution surface meshes to the computational grid. Weber et al. showed that basis functions in Bernstein-Bézier form yield a high quality embedding [WKS+11]. However, the presented approach did not make use of curved, isoparametric elements. Mezger et al. showed that isoparametric FE clearly improve the geometric approximation of coarse computational meshes [MTPS09]. They use a special meshing approach to make sure that all FE nodes lie on the surface mesh. If the geometry approximation of the computational grid is sufficiently close, this allows extrapolating the displacements to surface points outside the FE mesh without visible artefacts. A straight forward technique to avoid extrapolating displacements to points outside the FE mesh, is to completely submerge the high resolution surface mesh into the computational grid [LST09]. Unfortunately this approach is very inaccurate in comparison with boundary conforming FE meshes [ZSTB10].
The novel mapping scheme that will be presented in this work is motivated by developments in the field of shape editing techniques. There, both the pyramid coordinate scheme developed by Sheffer et al. as well as

the Green Coordinates introduced by Lipman et al. use a representation that includes the surface normal [SK04] [LLCO08].

3.4.5. Fast linear solvers

During the simulation, the linear system solve (and the update of the stiffness matrix if necessary) is the most expensive part of the simulation. Therefore, a fast linear solver is key to achieving real-time performance. Multigrid schemes have proven to be very efficient solvers. Consequently, it has been shown that deformable models can be efficiently solved using multigrid schemes on structured hexahedral grids [DGW11a]. Although this approach allows to simulate large models in real-time, a lot more degrees of freedom are necessary in comparison with boundary conforming unstructured FE grids [ZSTB10]. An alternative formulation that uses unstructured tetrahedral grids and transfer operators based on barycentric mapping was developed by Georgii et al. [GW08]. However, volume locking of linear tetrahedral elements can severely degrade the performance of this type of multigrid scheme.

3.4.6. GPU-based finite element solvers

It is especially challenging to run linear solvers on massively parallel hardware (graphic processing units - GPU). Allard et al. presented a matrix-free implementation of a GPU based conjugate gradient (CG) solver [ACF11]. Weber et al. used a novel GPU-compatible stiffness matrix assembly technique [WBS+12]. Although a pure CG solver can be very efficiently implemented on the GPU it can become very inefficient for higher resolution meshes if used without a preconditioner. However, only the simple Jacobi preconditioner can be readily used in a GPU framework. More powerful preconditioners such as incomplete Cholesky factorization (IC) or incomplete LU factorization (ILU) techniques are not only expensive to compute, but also have to be applied in a recursive fashion. An interesting alternative is the factorized sparse approximate inverse preconditioner (FSAI) [KY93]. This preconditioner is applied by a simple sparse matrix-vector multiplication (SpMV) which can be very efficiently carried out on the GPU. Its main drawback is the very high set-up time. In this work, we will present an approach to pre-compute the FSAI preconditioner and adopt a rotation warping scheme to adjust the preconditioner every time step. A similar scheme was previously proposed by Courtecuisse et al. [CAD+10].

3.4.7. Distributed computing

A possible solution for accelerating biomechanical simulations (especially if run in a context of a large CAS system) is the distribution of the computational workload over several workstations. Chrisochoides et al. showed how grid computing can help to reduce registration times during image guided neurosurgery [CFK+06]. However, for many interventions, the intraoperative navigation has to be updated in real-time (up to 25Hz). Thus, the question arises if distributed computing can actually speed up the image guidance in this scenario, or if the gain in processing power is offset by the additional delay for the inter-workstation communication. Several techniques have been developed for parallelizing applications over different computers. The message-passing interface (MPI) is used in high-performance computing on tightly coupled large-scale computer clusters [GLS99]. A much more flexible approach is offered by the common object request broker architecture (CORBA) [Vin97]. This standard allows exchanging data and remote method calls between programs written in different programming languages and running on different computers. However, this flexibility results in a complex architecture and difficult usage. The simple object access protocol (SOAP) relies on an XML message format to offer a simple, but very flexible access to distributed computing [BEK+00]. The drawback of this approach is that it is significantly slower than CORBA. This is due to the additional time that is required to parse the XML messages and the usage of the hypertext transfer protocol (HTTP).

3.5. Surgical cutting

Simulating surgical cuts with finite element based discretization techniques is a challenging problem. A straight forward approach is to simply remove the elements along the cutline [CDA00] [CJA+10]. However, this procedure does not only lead to a poor approximation of the cut, but it also violates the conservation of mass. In order to obtain a more accurate solution, local re-meshing around the cut has to be performed [MS97].

This approach can easily lead to ill-shaped tetrahedra (so called *sliver* elements) that can impair not only the performance, but also the stability of the simulation. Although complex procedures have been proposed that address this problem [BGTG04] [SDF07], the main drawbacks of the re-meshing approach still remains; the computationally demanding mesh adaptation procedure, the generation of many additional degrees of freedom as well as potential stability issues.
Novel methods thus seek to model the discontinuity in the solution without changing the grid topology. One possibility is to enrich the elements along the cutting front with additional, discontinuous basis functions. This approach is called the extended finite element method (X-FEM) [FB10]. Vigneron et al. use this method to compensate the *brain shift* that occurs during craniectomy in the presence of resected tissue [Vig09] [VWRV11]. In this scenario, a static linear elasticity model ist used. A first application of an X-FEM based technique for real-time cutting of 3D deformable objects was presented by Jerabkova et al. [JK09]. The work by Hegemann et al. showed how X-FEM based techniques can be used simulate complex fracture phenomena in the context of computer animation [HJST13]. Kaufmann et al. showed how the approach can be used to model very complex cuts through shell elements [KMB+09].
For 3D problems, there is currently no X-FEM based solution that allows for partially cutting elements along a progressing cutting front. This is not only a challenging geometric problem, but the numerical integration of partially cut elements is very difficult. Most importantly, harmonic shape functions have to be used if the cut ends within an element. As these functions do not have small, compact support as polygonal shape functions, it is necessary to enrich further elements in the neighborhood of the elements that are partially cut. An interesting solution to this problem was presented by Gracie et al. [GWB08]. The group used a technique based on the discontinuous Galerkin method [LNSO04] in order to couple enriched and non-enriched elements.
A different approach to the accurate simulation of surgical cutting is to use a hierarchical, high resolution hexahedral grid [JBB+10] [DGW11b]. The idea of this method is to simply model the cut by disconnecting the grid along the element boundaries. This simplifies not only the geometrical handling and the implementation of the cutting problem, but also enables the simulation of multiple cuts. Furthermore, the solution of the arising linear system of equations can be easily accelerated using

multigrid solvers due to the regular grid hierarchy. However, very high resolution grids have to be used in order to achieve a decent accuracy. Thus, the method needs much more degrees of freedom in comparison with X-FEM based techniques in order to achieve the same accuracy. One possibility to reduce the number of degrees of freedom is to group elements together in order to form so called composite elements [WDW13]. However, this procedure reduces the accuracy for corotated elasticity and fully non-linear formulations.

3.6. Validation of CAS systems

The validation of accuracy is a very important step towards a thorough evaluation for CAS systems [JGMJ06]. It is especially important for algorithms, modules and systems that are in a research or prototype state. In order to provide navigational information to the surgeon, CAS systems rely on suitable intraoperative sensors such as tracking systems, endoscopic video or ultrasound data. Typically, complex algorithms for sensor processing and registration techniques are used in order to align preoperative planning data to the patient based information provided by the sensors. In this context, the first validation step is to assess the accuracy of each individual component before proceeding to validate the whole system. Validation data can be acquired *in silico*, *in vitro* or *in vivo* including numerical simulations, phantoms or clinical data sets [JGMJ06].

Until now, numerical environments for *in silico* validation of sensor hardware and processing algorithms are usually restricted to simple synthetic data [HPE+07]. Even more elaborate approaches to sensor data simulation are often only used as a means for preliminary validation during development [RBS+12].

In contrast, phantom data is widely used for sensor processing validation. Models based on polyvinyl alcohol (PVA-C) can reproduce both the acoustic and the mechanical properties of human tissue and are suitable for validating ultrasound-based techniques [SAFP04]. The properties of the material can be tuned by changing the exact composition of the material and the number of cycles of a freeze-thaw process that is applied during manufacturing. Sufficient experience in handling this substance is required in order to accurately adjust its properties. Silicon

phantoms are often used in the context of endoscopic image processing. Examples include phantoms of the heart [RPL08], [SSPY10] and the liver [NME+09]. Different paints allow to emulate typical optical properties such as specular reflections. However, it is challenging to reproduce realistic texture patterns in this way.
Animal organs *in vitro* can also be used for accurate validation and benchmarking of image processing techniques in the context of endoscopic interventions [MHMB+13]. Careful planning and time consuming post processing is required in order to obtain ground truth values using this approach.
For the validation of non-rigid registration techniques it is important to obtain a sufficiently dense ground truth of the deformation field. This can be achieved by placing small marker balls inside a phantom [DCDM10]. Depending on the scenario, many marker balls are required for this purpose. Thus, it is important to set up the configuration in such a way that the processing of the ground truth data (segmentation, spatio-temporal registration) can be done (semi-)automatically. An important aspect in this application area is the accuracy of the phantom's mechanical behavior. Kerdok et al. performed the first quantitative analysis by means of force measurements and finite element analysis of appropriate silicon material for simple shapes [KCO+03]. More recent results show how phantoms for complex organ geometries can be constructed that provide an adequate accuracy in terms of the mechanical properties [HLBT12].

If people do not believe that mathematics is simple, it is only because they do not realize how complicated life is.
— John von Neumann

4. Biomechanical modeling of soft tissue

In this chapter the foundations of continuum mechanics based soft tissue modeling are introduced. We start by outlining the fundamentals of elasticity theory before presenting typical material models for biological soft tissue in general and the liver in particular. In order to facilitate the development of a real-time capable finite element models in the upcoming chapters, we finally present a simulation study that compares different model types with respect to their use for liver registration. The presentation of elasticity theory is kept as compact as possible without impairing accuracy or understandability. For more detailed treatments please refer to the excellent textbooks by Holzapfel [HG01] and Ogden [Ogd97].

4.1. A short introduction to elasticity

4.1.1. Kinematics

We consider a body $\mathcal{B}$ that can be viewed as a continuous distribution of matter in space and choose a standard right-handed orthonormal coordinate system as the reference frame (Fig. 4.1). The body moves in space from one instant of time to another, occupying different geometrical regions $\Omega_0,...,\Omega$ in the process. These regions are called configurations of $\mathcal{B}$ at time t. The configuration Ω_0 at time $t = 0$ is called the initial configuration while the configuration Ω at t is called the current configuration. Our goal is to describe the deformation of $\mathcal{B}$ with respect to a

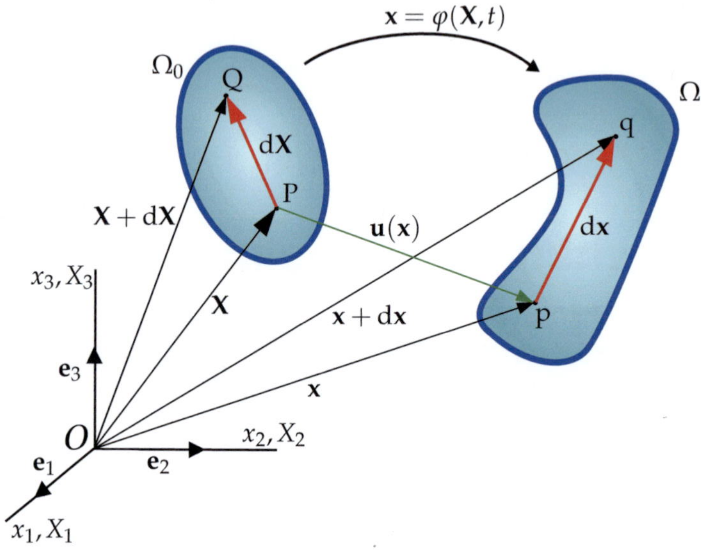

Figure 4.1.: Deformation of the body $\mathcal{B}$ with material points P, Q and infinitesimal line element $d\mathbf{X}$ from the reference configuration Ω_0 to the current configuration Ω (based on [Wik13])

reference configuration. Throughout this text, we will always assume the initial configuration to be our reference configuration.
We start by analyzing a continuum particle $\mathbf{P} \in \mathcal{B}$. It is important to note that $\mathbf{P}$ has no point mass (as opposed to a discrete particle in Newtonian mechanics). The particle is at position $\mathbf{X}$ in the reference configuration and moves to the position $\mathbf{x}$ in the current configuration (Fig. 4.1). We define the vector field

$$\mathbf{x} = \varphi(\mathbf{X}, t) \tag{4.1}$$

that maps the positions $\mathbf{X} \in \mathcal{B}$ of all points in the reference configuration to their respective positions $\mathbf{x}$ in the current configuration. In our analysis we assume that φ possess a continuous derivative and that it is uniquely invertible, i.e. the inverse mapping

$$\mathbf{X} = \varphi^{-1}(\mathbf{x}, t) \tag{4.2}$$

exists. Here, some important terminology should be introduced. φ is also called the motion of the body $\mathcal{B}$ over time. If we look at φ at a specific point in time, φ is called the deformation of the body. Thus, we speak of deformation if we mean the motion of a body that is independent of time. A body undergoing a deformation can change its shape, position and orientation. If the deformation is constant for all $\mathbf{X} \in \mathcal{B}$, the deformation consists only of translations and rotations and is called a rigid-body motion. Please note that in contrast to the common definition of deformation which implies changes to the body's shape, the continuum mechanics definition also includes rigid body motions.
Often the deformation is described in terms of the displacement

$$\mathbf{u}(\mathbf{X},t) = \mathbf{x}(\mathbf{X},t) - \mathbf{X} \tag{4.3}$$

of the body $\mathcal{B}$.
Continuum mechanics can be regarded as describing the behavior of infinitesimal line, area and volume elements during the passage from the reference to the current configuration. The second order tensor

$$\mathbf{F}(\mathbf{X},t) = \frac{\mathrm{d}\mathbf{x}}{\mathrm{d}\mathbf{X}} = \frac{\mathrm{d}x_i}{\mathrm{d}X_j} = x_{i,j} = \nabla\mathbf{x} = \mathrm{Grad}\mathbf{x} \tag{4.4}$$

describes the relation between the spatial line element $\mathrm{d}\mathbf{x}$ and the material line element $\mathrm{d}\mathbf{X}$ and is called the deformation gradient. Here, we showcased several different notations for the deformation gradient: The vectorial notation, the index notation and its shortened version as well as the notation using the nabla and the material gradient (Grad) operator. For more information on the notation of variables and operators used in this thesis please refer to the glossary. Using the relation (4.3), the deformation gradient can also be expressed in terms of the displacement field $\mathbf{u}(\mathbf{x},t)$:

$$\mathbf{F}(\mathbf{X},t) = \frac{\mathrm{d}\mathbf{u}}{\mathrm{d}\mathbf{X}} + \mathbf{I} = u_{i,j} + \delta_{ij} = \nabla\mathbf{u} + \mathbf{I} = \mathrm{Grad}\mathbf{u} + \mathbf{I} \tag{4.5}$$

Assuming that the derivative of the inverse mapping φ^{-1} exist, we can define the inverse of the deformation gradient

$$\mathbf{F}^{-1} = \frac{\mathrm{d}\mathbf{X}}{\mathrm{d}\mathbf{x}} = \mathrm{grad}\mathbf{X} \tag{4.6}$$

in an analogous manner. Please notice that the lowercase grad operator denotes the derivative with respect to $\mathbf{x}$ (spatial gradient).

4.1.2. Deformation of infinitesimal elements

In order to describe the change of infinitesimal volume elements due to deformation, we regard the parallelepiped that is spanned by the three non-coplanar line elements $d\mathbf{X}^{(1)}, d\mathbf{X}^{(2)}, d\mathbf{X}^{(3)}$ at the point $\mathbf{X}$ in $\mathcal{B}$. Assuming that this triad is positively oriented, its volume dV_0 in the reference configuration

$$dV_0 = (d\mathbf{X}^{(1)} \times d\mathbf{X}^{(2)}) \cdot d\mathbf{X}^{(3)} = \det(d\mathbf{X}^{(1)}, d\mathbf{X}^{(2)}, d\mathbf{X}^{(3)}) \tag{4.7}$$

is given by the triple scalar product. In accordance with eq. (4.4) we can write

$$d\mathbf{x}^{(i)} = \mathbf{F} d\mathbf{X}^{(i)} \tag{4.8}$$

and can thus derive the volume

$$dV = (d\mathbf{x}^{(1)} \times d\mathbf{x}^{(2)}) \cdot d\mathbf{x}^{(3)} = \det(\mathbf{F}d\mathbf{X}^{(1)}, \mathbf{F}d\mathbf{X}^{(2)}, \mathbf{F}d\mathbf{X}^{(3)}) \tag{4.9}$$

of the deformed element. Using the relationship

$$\det(\mathbf{AB}) = \det(\mathbf{A})\det(\mathbf{B}) \tag{4.10}$$

we can finally derive

$$dV = \det(\mathbf{F})\det(d\mathbf{X}^{(1)}, d\mathbf{X}^{(2)}, d\mathbf{X}^{(3)}) = \det(\mathbf{F})dV_0 \equiv J dV_0. \tag{4.11}$$

The determinant J of the deformation tensor (i.e. the Jacobian of the transformation φ) is the local ratio of current volume to reference volume of a material volume element. By definition (impenetrability of matter and non-singularity of $\mathbf{F}$),

$$J \equiv \det\mathbf{F} > 0. \tag{4.12}$$

It is also important to point out, especially in the context of soft tissue modeling, that for incompressible materials $J = 1$.
We now seek to describe the deformation of the infinitesimal surface element dA_0 with the normal $\mathbf{N}$ from its reference configuration $d\mathbf{A}_0 =$

$dA_0\mathbf{N}$ to its current configuration $d\mathbf{A} = dA\mathbf{n}$. We start by expressing the volume of a deformed parallelepiped eq. (4.9)

$$dV = d\mathbf{A} \cdot d\mathbf{x} = J dV_0 = J d\mathbf{A}_0 \cdot d\mathbf{X} \tag{4.13}$$

through its base area. Noting that

$$d\mathbf{A} \cdot d\mathbf{x} = d\mathbf{A} \cdot \mathbf{F} d\mathbf{X} = \mathbf{F}^T d\mathbf{A} \cdot d\mathbf{X}, \tag{4.14}$$

we can derive

$$\underbrace{(\mathbf{F}^T d\mathbf{A} - J d\mathbf{A}_0)}_{0} \cdot d\mathbf{X} = 0 \tag{4.15}$$

As this must hold for arbitrary line elements $d\mathbf{X}$, we can describe the deformation of the arbitrary surface element $d\mathbf{A}_0$ through the deformation gradient tensor $\mathbf{F}$:

$$d\mathbf{A} = J\mathbf{F}^{-T} d\mathbf{A}_0 \tag{4.16}$$

This relationship is known as Nanson's formula.

4.1.3. Strain measures

The deformation gradient tensor characterizes the deformation of infinitesimal line, area and volume elements during the body motion. In order to construct meaningful material laws it is necessary to determine the strain (i.e. the 3D equivalent of stretch) inside a body. Strain can be described as a measure for the change in length of infinitesimal line elements. It should be pointed out that strain is not a necessarily a physically measurable quantity, but rather a theoretical concept. Consequently, many different strain measures exist. In the following, the most important strain tensors for soft tissue modeling are presented.
First, it is important to understand that the deformation gradient tensor is not a suitable strain tensor; this can be seen from the polar decomposition theorem.

Theorem 1 *The polar decomposition theorem: For any non-singular second order tensor* $\mathbf{A}$ *there exist a unique symmetric, positive definite second order tensor* $\mathbf{U}$ *and an orthogonal second-order tensor* $\mathbf{R}$ *such that*

$$\mathbf{A} = \mathbf{R}\mathbf{U} \tag{4.17}$$

For a proof we refer to Ogden [Ogd97]. With respect to the deformation gradient tensor (keep in mind that it is non-singular) this means that it can be decomposed into a pure rotation matrix $\mathbf{R}$ and a pure stretch matrix $\mathbf{U}$. Thus, $\mathbf{F}$ changes under pure rigid body motions. For apparent reasons, the invariance under rigid body motions is an important property of a useful strain measure. Thus $\mathbf{F}$ cannot be directly used as a strain tensor. One possibility to recover rotational invariance is to perform a polar decomposition for each computation step and to use the remaining stretch matrix as a strain measure. Alternatively, a quadratic strain measure can be used. The first approach is often used in real-time simulations (see chapter 5), while the second possibility is used in classical solid mechanics as it allows for a better analytic analysis of the ensuing equations.
Upon inserting the deformation gradient tensor into the Cauchy-Green strain tensor

$$\mathbf{C} = \mathbf{F}^T\mathbf{F} \tag{4.18}$$

it is easy to see that $\mathbf{C}$ is rotation invariant (keep in mind that $\mathbf{R}^T\mathbf{R} = \mathbf{I}$ due to the orthogonality of $\mathbf{R}$):

$$\mathbf{C} = \mathbf{F}^T\mathbf{F} = (\mathbf{RU})^T\mathbf{RU} = \mathbf{U}^T\mathbf{R}^T\mathbf{RU} = \mathbf{U}^T\mathbf{U}. \tag{4.19}$$

Another important strain measure is the related Green-Lagrange strain tensor

$$\mathbf{E} = \frac{1}{2}(\mathbf{C} - \mathbf{I}) = \frac{1}{2}(\mathbf{F}^T\mathbf{F} - \mathbf{I}) = \frac{1}{2}((\nabla\mathbf{u} + \mathbf{I})^T(\nabla\mathbf{u} + \mathbf{I}) - \mathbf{I}), \tag{4.20}$$

which is also symmetric and rotation invariant. Please note that both tensors are non-linear and must be in order to be rotation invariant. In order to facilitate the development of linear elasticity theory later on, we list the infinitesimal strain tensor

$$\epsilon = \frac{1}{2}(\nabla\mathbf{u} + \nabla\mathbf{u}^T), \tag{4.21}$$

which is the linearization of the Green-Lagrange strain tensor.

4.1.4. Balance principles

In classical continuum mechanics, the behavior of objects is governed by four conservation laws: The conservation of mass, the balance of linear and angular momentum as well as the conservation of energy.

It is intuitively clear, that the body $\mathcal{B}$ is a closed system and its mass m does not change, even if $\mathcal{B}$ does occupy different geometrical regions $\Omega_0,...,\Omega$ over time. If we denote the density of $\mathcal{B}$ with $\rho_0(\mathbf{X})$ in the reference configuration and the density in the current configuration with $\rho(\mathbf{x})$ we thus require the mass to be the same in the current and in the reference configuration:

$$m = \int_{\Omega_0} \rho_0(\mathbf{X})\mathrm{dV}_0 = \int_{\Omega} \rho(\mathbf{x})\mathrm{dV} = \text{const.} > 0 \tag{4.22}$$

This is the conservation of mass in integral form. The linear momentum in the current configuration

$$\int_{\Omega} \rho\mathbf{v}\mathrm{dV} = \int_{\Omega} \rho\dot{\mathbf{x}}\mathrm{dV} \tag{4.23}$$

is changed, when $\mathcal{B}$ is subjected to external forces. In this context, so called volumetric body forces (e.g. gravity, electromagnetic forces) are distinguished from contact forces that act on the surface of $\mathcal{B}$. The gravitational body force

$$\int_{\Omega} \rho\mathbf{g}\mathrm{dV} \tag{4.24}$$

can be written in its integral form using the gravitational constant $\mathbf{g}$. An analogous integral description for the contact force

$$\int_{\partial\Omega} \mathbf{t}(\mathbf{x},\partial\Omega)\mathrm{d}\mathbf{A} \tag{4.25}$$

can be found by defining the contact force density (or surface traction vector) $\mathbf{t}(\mathbf{x},\partial\Omega)$. The balance of linear momentum can be written as

$$\int_{\partial\Omega} \mathbf{t}(\mathbf{x},\partial\Omega)\mathrm{d}\mathbf{A} + \int_{\Omega} \rho\mathbf{g}\mathrm{dV} \equiv \frac{\mathrm{D}}{\mathrm{Dt}} \int_{\Omega} \rho\mathbf{v}\mathrm{dV} = \int_{\Omega} \rho\dot{\mathbf{v}}\mathrm{dV}. \tag{4.26}$$

For a body to be in complete equilibrium it is not sufficient that all internal and external forces acting on the body are in balance. Even if all external forces cancel out (static equilibrium) the body can still be subjected to a rotational motion, if these forces act on different points of the body. The rotational equilibrium is ensured by the balance of rotational momentum. By using the position vector $\mathbf{r}(\mathbf{x}) = \mathbf{x} - \mathbf{x}_0$ relative to a fixed point $\mathbf{x}_0$ it can be formulated as

$$\int_{\partial\Omega} \mathbf{r} \times \mathbf{t}(\mathbf{x},\partial\Omega)\mathrm{d}\mathbf{A} + \int_{\Omega} \mathbf{r} \times \rho\mathbf{g}\mathrm{dV} \equiv \frac{\mathrm{D}}{\mathrm{Dt}} \int_{\Omega} \mathbf{r} \times \rho\mathbf{v}\mathrm{dV} = \int_{\Omega} \mathbf{r} \times \rho\dot{\mathbf{v}}\mathrm{dV}. \tag{4.27}$$

In the context of thermodynamics the conservation of energy and the balance of momentum is supplemented by the conservation of energy. However, in the realm of soft tissue simulation the thermal effects of the body motion are extremely small and are usually neglected. Thus, the body motion can be fully described using the three balance principles described above.

4.1.5. The concept of stress

Cauchy postulated that the surface traction vector $\mathbf{t}$ has the same value for all boundaries with the same normal direction $\mathbf{n}$. In other words, $\mathbf{t}$ only depends on the surface normal and we can write:

$$\mathbf{t}(\mathbf{x},\partial\Omega) = \mathbf{t}(\mathbf{x},\mathbf{n}). \tag{4.28}$$

From this postulate, Cauchy's fundamental stress theorem can be established.

Theorem 2 *Cauchy's stress theorem: Provided that it is continuous in* $\mathbf{x}$*, the stress vector* $\mathbf{t}(\mathbf{x},\mathbf{n})$ *depends linearly on* $\mathbf{n}$*, i.e. there exists a second order tensor field* σ *independent of* $\mathbf{n}$*, such that*

$$\mathbf{t}(\mathbf{x},\mathbf{n}) = \sigma(\mathbf{x})\mathbf{n} \tag{4.29}$$

for all $\mathbf{x}$ *in* $\mathcal{B}$*. The tensor* σ *is called the Cauchy stress (or true stress) tensor.*

The theorem is usually proven ([Ogd97], [Bon97]) by constructing a tetrahedron that lies in the Cartesian rectangular planes (see Fig. 4.2). After applying the balance of linear momentum eq. (4.26) and collapsing the height of the triangle ($h \mapsto 0$) the external body and inertia forces vanish. The application of the postulate then leads to Cauchy's stress tensor. Furthermore, it can be shown that the balance of rotational momentum implies the symmetry of the Cauchy stress tensor [HG01].

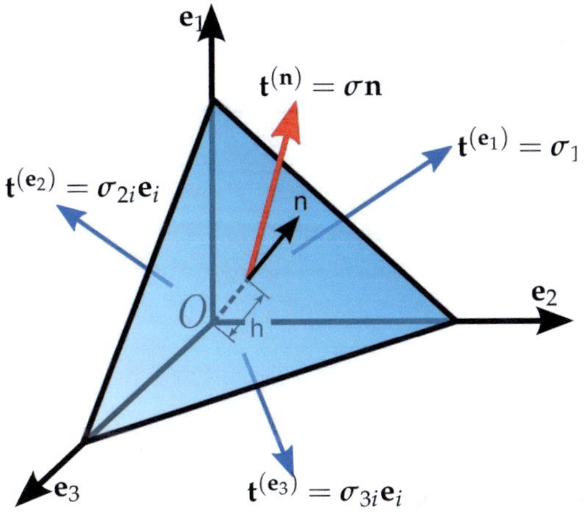

Figure 4.2.: Cauchy's tetrahedron: The traction $\mathbf{t}^{(\mathbf{n})}$ on the surface with normal $\mathbf{n}$ can be expressed as a linear combination of the tractions on the coordinate planes (based on [Wik13]).

As a direct consequence we can express the force

$$\mathbf{df} = \mathbf{t}(\sigma, \mathbf{n})\mathrm{d}\mathbf{A} = \sigma(\mathbf{x})\mathbf{n}\mathrm{dA} \tag{4.30}$$

on an infinitesimal surface element (the so called surface tractions) in the current configuration using the Cauchy stress tensor and the surface normal.
Please note that the balance laws have so far been formulated in the current, deformed configuration. However, in a typical scenario the deformed geometry of $\mathcal{B}$ is actually the solution that we would like to solve for. It is thus impossible to integrate over the current configuration. This problem can be overcome by relating all forces to the reference configuration and solving the problem using the so called material description. In order to facilitate this formulation, we relate the surface force $\mathbf{df}$ to the undeformed surface element $\mathrm{d}\mathbf{A}_0$ through the use of Nanson's formula eq. (4.16):

$$\mathbf{df} = \sigma(\mathbf{x})\mathbf{n}\mathrm{dA} = \sigma J\mathbf{F}^{-T}\mathbf{N}\mathrm{dA}_0 = \mathbf{PN}\mathrm{dA}_0 \tag{4.31}$$

Here, we introduced the first Piola-Kirchhoff stress tensor

$$\mathbf{P} = J\sigma\mathbf{F}^{-T} \tag{4.32}$$

which relates surface forces in the current configuration to surface elements in the reference configuration. The passage from σ to $\mathbf{P}$ is often referred to as the Piola transformation. Please note that, in contrast to the Cauchy stress tensor, the first Piola-Kirchhoff tensor is not symmetric (because $\mathbf{F}$ is generally not symmetric).
Many different stress measures have been proposed in the literature apart from the Cauchy and the first Piola-Kirchhoff stress tensor. At this point we will only mention the symmetric second Piola-Kirchoff stress tensor

$$\mathbf{S} = J\mathbf{F}^{-1}\sigma\mathbf{F}^{-T} = \mathbf{F}^{-1}\mathbf{P} = \mathbf{S}^{T} \tag{4.33}$$

which is very important in the context of soft tissue simulations for reasons that will be extensively discussed in chapter 4.2.

4.1.6. Boundary value problem of elasticity

The conservations laws can be combined into a single partial differential equation (PDE). Together with appropriate boundary conditions and a material law, this PDE forms a boundary value problem. We start by inserting the Cauchy stress tensor into the balance of linear momentum (eq. 4.26) to derive

$$\int_{\partial\Omega} \sigma(\mathbf{x})\mathbf{n}\mathrm{dA} + \int_{\Omega} \rho\mathbf{g}\mathrm{dV} = \int_{\Omega} \rho\dot{\mathbf{v}}\mathrm{dV}. \tag{4.34}$$

From this, Cauchy's first equation of motion

$$\int_{\Omega} \mathrm{div}\sigma(\mathbf{x})\mathrm{dV} + \int_{\Omega} \rho\mathbf{g}\mathrm{dV} = \int_{\Omega} \rho\dot{\mathbf{v}}\mathrm{dV} \tag{4.35}$$

is derived by applying the divergence theorem (A.1.1) to the surface term. As this relation has to hold for any volume dV in $\mathcal{B}$ the differential (local) form

$$\mathrm{div}\sigma(\mathbf{x}) + \rho\mathbf{g} = \rho\dot{\mathbf{v}} \tag{4.36}$$

immediately follows from the integral (global) form (4.35).

As stated above, this partial differential equation cannot be solved when formulated in terms of the current (unknown) configuration (spatial description). Therefore, we use the mass conservation and Nanson's formula to express eq. (4.34) with respect to the reference configuration:

$$\int_{\partial\Omega_0} \sigma J \mathbf{F}^{-T} \mathbf{N} \mathrm{d}\mathbf{A}_0 + \int_{\Omega_0} \rho_0 \mathbf{g} \mathrm{dV}_0 = \int_{\Omega_0} \rho_0 \dot{\mathbf{v}} \mathrm{dV}_0. \tag{4.37}$$

Inserting the definition of the first Piola-Kirchhoff stress tensor eq. (4.32) and application of the divergence theorem yields the material description of Cauchy's first equation of motion

$$\int_{\Omega_0} \mathrm{Div}\mathbf{P} \mathrm{dV}_0 + \int_{\Omega_0} \rho_0 \mathbf{g} \mathrm{dV}_0 = \int_{\Omega_0} \rho_0 \dot{\mathbf{v}} \mathrm{dV}_0. \tag{4.38}$$

The boundary value problem is typically stated using the local formulation

$$\mathrm{Div}\mathbf{P} + \rho_0 \mathbf{g} = \rho_0 \dot{\mathbf{v}} \qquad \forall \mathbf{x} \in \Omega_0 \tag{4.39}$$

of Cauchy's equation of motion in material description. In addition to the equilibrium equation, boundary conditions have to be specified on the elastic body $\mathcal{B}$ in order to pose a physically sensible problem (please see Fig. 4.3 for an example). The parts of the surface $\Gamma_D \subseteq \partial\Omega$ where the position (or the displacement) of the body are known are called Dirichlet boundary conditions. In contrast, surface tractions are imposed on the Neumann boundary Γ_N. In order for the problem to be well posed, either Dirichlet or Neumann boundary conditions have to be prescribed on the whole boundary ($\partial\Omega = \Gamma_D \cup \Gamma_N$). Furthermore, Γ_D and Γ_N are not allowed to overlap, i.e. $\Gamma_D \cap \Gamma_N = \emptyset$. By specifying the spaces of functions that satisfy these boundary conditions

$$V_D(\Gamma_D, \overline{\mathbf{x}}) = \{\mathbf{x} | \mathbf{x} = \overline{\mathbf{x}} \qquad \forall \mathbf{x} \in \Gamma_D\} \tag{4.40}$$

$$V_N(\Gamma_N, \overline{\mathbf{t}}) = \{\mathbf{x} | (\sigma \mathbf{n}) = \overline{\mathbf{t}} \qquad \forall \mathbf{x} \in \Gamma_N\} \tag{4.41}$$

we can finally state the boundary value problem of non-linear elasticity: Find $\mathbf{x} \in C^2(\Omega) \cap C^1(\overline{\Omega}) \cap V_D(\Gamma_D, \overline{\mathbf{x}}) \cap V_N(\Gamma_N, \overline{\mathbf{t}})$ s.t. eq. 4.39 holds.

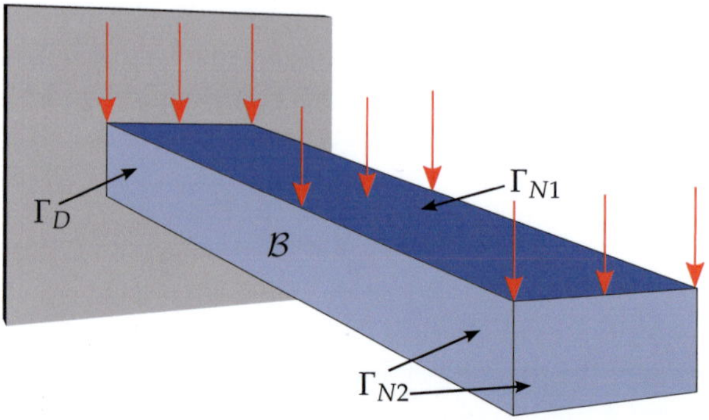

Figure 4.3.: A cantilever beam is fixed at the left end (zero displacement at Dirichlet boundary Γ_D) and a uniform surface pressure is applied at the top (on Neumann boundary Γ_{N1}). Zero force boundary conditions are prescribed on all other surfaces (Neumann boundary Γ_{N2}).

4.2. Material laws for biological soft tissue

The boundary value problem introduced in the previous section cannot be solved without a constitutive equation that relates the position $\mathbf{x}$ (or the displacement $\mathbf{u}$) to the stress tensor values. In the context of elastic bodies this relationship is called the response function $\mathcal{G}(\mathbf{F}(\mathbf{X},t),\mathbf{X})$. In the following section we will see that some of the already encountered strain and stress measures form special (so called work conjugate) pairs. The work conjugancy relationship arises from the definition of the internal elastic energy that is stored in $\mathcal{B}$ during the deformation. Furthermore we will see that the internal elastic energy is an important concept in the context of hyperelastic material models, which are the most important class of non-linear models for soft tissue mechanics. We will also introduce basic techniques for modeling viscoelastic behavior. Finally, it is shown under which assumptions the nonlinear elasticity problem reduces to a linear problem.

4.2.1. Mechanical energy in elastic bodies

If the material response is purely elastic and no energy is dissipated as heat, the balance of mechanical energy can be directly derived from the equation of motion. Multiplying Cauchy's equation of motion (4.36) with the velocity $\mathbf{v}$ yields

$$\mathrm{div}\sigma \cdot \mathbf{v} + \rho \mathbf{g} \cdot \mathbf{v} = \rho \dot{\mathbf{v}} \cdot \mathbf{v}. \tag{4.42}$$

By using the product rule (see A.1.2) and introducing the spatial velocity gradient $\mathbf{l} = \mathrm{grad}\mathbf{v}$ we derive

$$\mathrm{div}(\sigma \mathbf{v}) - \sigma : \mathbf{l} + \rho \mathbf{g} \cdot \mathbf{v} = \rho \dot{\mathbf{v}} \cdot \mathbf{v}. \tag{4.43}$$

We note that in light of the product differentiation rule, the mass term can be rewritten to

$$\rho \dot{\mathbf{v}} \cdot \mathbf{v} = \rho \frac{1}{2} \overline{\mathbf{v} \cdot \mathbf{v}}^{\,\cdot} = \rho \frac{\mathrm{D}}{\mathrm{Dt}} \frac{1}{2} \mathbf{v}^2. \tag{4.44}$$

The spatial velocity gradient $\mathbf{l}$ is usually additively decomposed

$$\mathbf{l} = \mathbf{d} + \mathbf{w} \tag{4.45}$$

into the symmetric rate of deformation tensor

$$\mathbf{d} = \frac{1}{2}(\mathbf{l} + \mathbf{l}^T) = \mathbf{d}^T \tag{4.46}$$

and the antisymmetric rate of rotation sensor

$$\mathbf{w} = \frac{1}{2}(\mathbf{l} - \mathbf{l}^T) = -\mathbf{w}^T. \tag{4.47}$$

It is quickly shown that the material velocity gradient

$$\mathrm{Grad}\mathbf{v} = \frac{\partial \mathbf{v}(\mathbf{X},t)}{\partial \mathbf{X}} = \frac{\mathrm{D}}{\mathrm{Dt}} \frac{\partial \varphi(\mathbf{X},t)}{\partial \mathbf{X}} = \dot{\mathbf{F}} \tag{4.48}$$

is identical to the time rate change $\dot{\mathbf{F}}$ of the deformation gradient. The relationship between the spatial velocity gradient $\mathbf{l}$ and $\dot{\mathbf{F}}$ is given by

$$\mathbf{l} = \frac{\partial \mathbf{v}}{\partial \mathbf{x}} = \frac{\mathrm{D}}{\mathrm{Dt}} \frac{\partial \varphi\ (\mathbf{X},t)}{\partial \mathbf{x}} = \frac{\mathrm{D}}{\mathrm{Dt}} \frac{\partial \varphi\ (\mathbf{X},t)}{\partial \mathbf{X}} \frac{\partial \mathbf{X}}{\partial \mathbf{x}} = \dot{\mathbf{F}}\mathbf{F}^{-1}. \tag{4.49}$$

We note that due to the symmetry of σ, we have

$$\sigma : \mathbf{l} = \sigma : \mathbf{d} + \sigma : \mathbf{w} = \sigma : \mathbf{d}. \tag{4.50}$$

Inserting this result into eq. (4.43) as well as using the relationship (4.45) and subsequently integrating over the volume of the current configuration yields

$$\frac{\mathrm{D}}{\mathrm{Dt}}\int_{\Omega}\frac{1}{2}\rho\mathbf{v}^2\mathrm{dV} + \int_{\Omega}\sigma : \mathbf{d}\mathrm{dV} = \int_{\Omega}\mathrm{div}(\sigma\mathbf{v})\mathrm{dV} + \int_{\Omega}\rho\mathbf{g}\cdot\mathbf{v}\mathrm{dV}. \tag{4.51}$$

The balance equation for mechanical energy in spatial description

$$\frac{\mathrm{D}}{\mathrm{Dt}}\int_{\Omega}\frac{1}{2}\rho\mathbf{v}^2\mathrm{dV} + \int_{\Omega}\sigma : \mathbf{d}\mathrm{dV} = \int_{\partial\Omega}\mathbf{t}\cdot\mathbf{v}\mathrm{dA} + \int_{\Omega}\rho\mathbf{g}\cdot\mathbf{v}\mathrm{dV} \tag{4.52}$$

immediately follows from the application of the divergence theorem and the definition of the surface traction (4.30). The right hand side of the equilibrium equation is the external mechanical power or rate of external mechanical work

$$\mathcal{P}_{ext}(t) = \int_{\partial\Omega}\mathbf{t}\cdot\mathbf{v}\mathrm{d}\mathbf{A} + \int_{\Omega}\rho\mathbf{g}\cdot\mathbf{v}\mathrm{dV} \tag{4.53}$$

is the power input on the region Ω. The kinetic energy

$$\mathcal{K}(t) = \int_{\Omega}\frac{1}{2}\rho\mathbf{v}^2\mathrm{dV} \tag{4.54}$$

can be regarded as an generalization of Newtonian mechanics to continuum mechanics. If $\mathcal{K}$ is zero (i.e. no inertia forces), then the dynamic BVP reduces to a non-linear static problem. The stress power or rate of internal mechanical work is given by

$$\mathcal{P}_{int}(t) = \int_{\Omega}\sigma : \mathbf{d}\mathrm{dV}. \tag{4.55}$$

In order to derive the balance of mechanical energy in material (Lagrangian) form, we formulate the internal mechanical work in terms of the material description:

$$\mathcal{P}_{int}(t) = \int_{\Omega_0} \sigma : \mathbf{l} J \mathrm{dV}_0 = \int_{\Omega_0} J\sigma : \dot{\mathbf{F}}\mathbf{F}^{-1} \mathrm{dV}_0 = \int_{\Omega_0} J \mathrm{tr}(\sigma^T \dot{\mathbf{F}}\mathbf{F}^{-1}) \mathrm{dV}_0 \tag{4.56}$$

$$= \int_{\Omega_0} J \mathrm{tr}(\dot{\mathbf{F}}\mathbf{F}^{-1}\sigma) \mathrm{dV}_0 = \int_{\Omega_0} J \mathrm{tr}((\dot{\mathbf{F}}\mathbf{F}^{-1}\sigma)^T) \mathrm{dV}_0 \tag{4.57}$$

$$= \int_{\Omega_0} J \mathrm{tr}(\sigma^T \mathbf{F}^{-T} \dot{\mathbf{F}}^T) \mathrm{dV}_0 = \int_{\Omega_0} J\sigma\mathbf{F}^{-T} : \dot{\mathbf{F}} \mathrm{dV}_0 = \int_{\Omega_0} \mathbf{P} : \dot{\mathbf{F}} \mathrm{dV}_0 \tag{4.58}$$

We furthermore define the first Piola-Kirchhoff traction vector

$$\mathbf{T} \mathrm{d}\mathbf{A}_0 = \mathbf{t} \mathrm{d}\mathbf{A} \tag{4.59}$$

in order establish the balance of mechanical energy in material description:

$$\frac{\mathrm{D}}{\mathrm{Dt}} \int_{\Omega_0} \frac{1}{2} \rho_0 \mathbf{v}^2 \mathrm{dV}_0 + \int_{\Omega_0} \mathbf{P} : \dot{\mathbf{F}} \mathrm{dV}_0 = \int_{\partial\Omega_0} \mathbf{T} \cdot \mathbf{v} \mathrm{d}\mathbf{A}_0 + \int_{\Omega_0} \rho_0 \mathbf{g} \cdot \mathbf{v} \mathrm{dV}_0 \tag{4.60}$$

The stress power per unit reference volume

$$w_{int} = J\sigma : \mathbf{d} = \mathbf{P} : \dot{\mathbf{F}} = \mathbf{S} : \dot{\mathbf{E}} \tag{4.61}$$

of a material is thus given by the double contraction of a stress tensor and an associated strain rate tensor. The equation above lists the most important ones of these couples known as work conjugate pairs (please refer to the appendix A.2 on how to derive the work conjugacy of the second Piola-Kirchhoff stress tensor $\mathbf{S}$ and the material time derivative of the Green-Lagrange strain tensor $\dot{\mathbf{E}}$).

4.2.2. Hyperelastic materials

Biological soft tissue is usually modeled using a phenomenological approach. Based on *in vitro* or *in vivo* measurements, mathematical models

are fitted to experimental data that describe the stress-strain relationship. In this section, the important hyperelastic approach to soft tissue modeling is discussed. Although only isotropic hyperelastic materials are considered at this point, the approach can be extended to include anisotropic material behavior [HG01]. The extension of the model to viscoelastic material response is detailed in the subsequent section.
Materials are called Cauchy-elastic if the stress field in the deformed configuration only depends on the state of deformation and not on the deformation history. That means we can define a so called response function $\mathcal{G}$ that relates the deformation gradient tensor $\mathbf{F}$ to the Cauchy stress field σ:

$$\sigma(\mathbf{x},t) = \mathcal{G}(\mathbf{F}(\mathbf{X},t),\mathbf{X}) \tag{4.62}$$

By inserting this definition into the already familiar Piola transformation

$$\mathbf{P} = J\sigma\mathbf{F}^{-T} = J\mathcal{G}(\mathbf{F})\mathbf{F}^{-T} = \mathcal{H}(\mathbf{F}) \tag{4.63}$$

we can define the response function $\mathcal{H}$ that relates the deformation to the first Piola-Kirchhoff stress tensor.
The problem of describing a suitable response function for biological soft tissue is usually tackled by describing the internal energy of a material. For this purpose, we postulate the existence of a so called elastic potential or strain energy function Ψ that is defined per unit reference volume. Materials for which Ψ exists and only depends on the deformation ($\Psi = \Psi(\mathbf{F})$) and not on the deformation history are called (pure) hyperelastic materials.
We now show how elastic response functions for work conjugate stress-strain tensors pairs can be derived from the elastic potential. The time derivative of the internal energy

$$\dot{\Psi} = w_{int} = \mathbf{P} : \dot{\mathbf{F}} \tag{4.64}$$

is the internal work which can be expressed through the work conjugate pair. On the other hand, we can apply the chain rule to derive

$$\dot{\Psi} = \frac{\partial \Psi}{\partial \mathbf{F}} : \dot{\mathbf{F}}. \tag{4.65}$$

By subtracting the above equations we obtain

$$\left(\frac{\partial\Psi}{\partial\mathbf{F}} - \mathbf{P}\right) : \dot{\mathbf{F}} = 0 \tag{4.66}$$

which has to hold for arbitrary $\mathbf{F}$ and $\dot{\mathbf{F}}$ and thus we can conclude:

$$\mathbf{P} = \frac{\partial\Psi}{\partial\mathbf{F}} = \mathcal{H}(\mathbf{F}) \tag{4.67}$$

The same technique can be used to express the second Piola-Kirchhoff stress tensor

$$\mathbf{S} = \frac{\partial\Psi}{\partial\mathbf{E}} = \mathcal{H}(\mathbf{E}) \tag{4.68}$$

in terms of the Green-Lagrange strain tensor. This relationship allows to compute the response function once the relationship between the elastic potential and the deformation is known. Please note that while hyperelastic materials (also called Green-elastic) are evidently always Cauchy-elastic, the converse is not necessarily true. Although the stress field for Cauchy-elastic materials is independent of the deformation path, in contrast to hyperleastic materials the work done (i.e. the internal energy) by the stress field can depend on the deformation history.
Naturally, material models should be constructed in a way that the boundary value problem has an (ideally unique) solution that corresponds to the physical observations. The mathematical treatment of the uniqueness and existence of non-linear elasticity problems is still an area of active research and revolves around the concept of the polyconvexity of strain-energy functions (see e.g. [HN03] [H$^+$94]).
On the physical level, there is one important necessary condition for the strain energy function: It should be invariant under superimposed rigid-body motions, i.e.

$$\Psi(\mathbf{F}) = \Psi(\mathbf{QF}) \tag{4.69}$$

for all orthogonal tensors $\mathbf{Q}$. If we choose $\mathbf{Q}$ to be the transpose of the orthogonal rotation tensor $\mathbf{R}$ that arises from the polar decomposition (see theorem 1) of $\mathbf{F}$,

$$\Psi(\mathbf{F}) = \Psi(\mathbf{R}^T\mathbf{R}\mathbf{U}) = \Psi(\mathbf{U}) \tag{4.70}$$

we learn that Ψ has to be independent from the rotational component $\mathbf{R}$ in order to be invariant under superimposed rigid-body motions. In

classical continuum mechanics, the strain energy is usually expressed in terms of the quadratic, rotation invariant Cauchy-Green deformation tensor $\mathbf{C}$ (or the Green-Lagrange tensor $\mathbf{E}$) instead of the pure stretch tensor $\mathbf{U}$. Thus it is not necessary to perform a polar decomposition during analysis.
A material is called isotropic if its properties (e.g. the stress response) are identical in all directions. This means, that the property is not affected if the reference configuration is translated or rotated. If the strain energy function is formulated in terms of the Cauchy-Green deformation tensor $\mathbf{C}$, this requirement can be expressed mathematically as

$$\Psi(\mathbf{C}) = \Psi(\mathbf{Q}\mathbf{C}\mathbf{Q}^T) \tag{4.71}$$

where $\mathbf{Q}^T$ again denotes an arbitrary orthogonal tensor (rotation matrix). The representation theorem of invariants shows how to construct the strain energy function for isotropic materials [Hol00]:

Theorem 3 *The representation theorem for invariants: If a scalar-valued tensor function with the argument* $\mathbf{C}$ *is an invariant under a rotation according to (4.71), it may be expressed in terms of the principal invariants of* $\mathbf{C}$*:*

$$I_1(\mathbf{C}) = \mathrm{tr}\mathbf{C} \tag{4.72}$$

$$I_2(\mathbf{C}) = \frac{1}{2}\left[(\mathrm{tr}\mathbf{C})^2 - \mathrm{tr}(\mathbf{C})^2\right] \tag{4.73}$$

$$I_3(\mathbf{C}) = \det\mathbf{C} \tag{4.74}$$

The questions remains how the strain energy function should be constructed. If Ψ is continuously differentiable with respect to the invariants, we can expand Ψ into the infinite power series

$$\Psi(I_1, I_2, I_3) = \sum_{p,g,r=0}^{\infty} c_{pgr}(I_1 - 3)^p (I_2 - 3)^q (I_3 - 1)^r. \tag{4.75}$$

Here, the coefficients c_{pqr} are the material parameters that have to be experimentally determined. Please note that this expansion has been chosen such that the material is energy-free in the reference configuration (i.e. $\mathbf{C} = \mathbf{I}$). It is a common approach to separate the strain energy functional

$$\Psi = \Psi_{iso} + \Psi_{vol} \tag{4.76}$$

into a part Ψ_{vol} that only depends on the volume change and a so called isochoric part Ψ_{iso} that is independent of the volumetric changes [Hol00].
We have already discovered in section 4.1.2 that $I_3 = \det\mathbf{C} = (\det\mathbf{F})^2$ is a measure of the volumetric change during the deformation. Therefore, it is readily seen that the general expression

$$\Psi_{vol} = \sum_{r=0}^{\infty} c_r (I_3 - 1)^r \tag{4.77}$$

describes an internal energy that is induced by volumetric changes. A simple and yet widely used formulation is

$$\Psi_{vol} = p(I_3 - 1)^2. \tag{4.78}$$

In the fully incompressible case, p serves a Lagrange multiplier during the computation of the solution and can be associated with the hydrostatic pressure. In this case, p is not a material parameter, but can be determined through the incompressibility constraint. If the material is modeled as nearly incompressible (which is often the case for biological soft tissue), p can be regarded as a penalty factor for the volumetric change. In this case, it is often replaced through its inverse $D_1 = 1/p$.
If the material is incompressible, there are no volume changes and the isochoric part of the strain energy

$$\Psi_{iso}(\mathbf{C}) = \Psi_{iso}(I_1, I_2) \tag{4.79}$$

depends on the invariants I_1, I_2. However, these invariants vary during volumetric changes. In the context of compressible materials, the modified deformation tensor $\overline{\mathbf{F}} = J^{-1/3}\mathbf{F}$ and the associated modified right Cauchy-Green tensor $\overline{\mathbf{C}} = \overline{\mathbf{F}}^T\overline{\mathbf{F}}$ are used as deformation measures in the strain energy function. It is evident, that $\det\overline{\mathbf{F}} = \det\overline{\mathbf{C}} = 1$ and thus the strain energy

$$\Psi_{iso}(\overline{\mathbf{C}}) = \Psi_{iso}(\overline{I}_1, \overline{I}_2) \tag{4.80}$$

based on the invariants $\overline{I}_1, \overline{I}_2$ of $\overline{\mathbf{C}}$ is not influenced by volumetric changes.
In the following section, common material models are presented for the isochoric strain energy. Although we will formulate them for the

incompressible case in the form of the potential $\Psi_{iso}(\mathbf{C})$, it is important to note that they generalize to the compressible domain by simply using the modified formulation $\Psi_{iso}(\overline{\mathbf{C}})$ based on the modified deformation measures introduced above [Hol00].
The Mooney-Rivlin material model

$$\Psi_{iso}(\mathbf{C}) = c_1(I_1 - 3) + c_2(I_2 - 3) \tag{4.81}$$

has originally been developed for isotropic rubber-like materials and is often used for soft tissue modeling. One of the simplest hyperelastic models is the neo-Hookean model

$$\Psi_{iso}(\mathbf{C}) = c_1(I_1 - 3). \tag{4.82}$$

The material parameter c_1 can be associated with the shear modulus μ by the formula $\mu = 2c_1$. The neo-Hookean model can be considered a special case of the reduced polynomial model

$$\Psi_{iso}(\mathbf{C}) = \sum_{i=1}^{N} c_i(I_1 - 3)^i \tag{4.83}$$

with $N = 1$ [RES10].
The simplest model for a compressible hyperelastic material is the Saint Venant-Kirchhoff model. For simplicity reasons, its strain energy function

$$\Psi(\mathbf{E}) = \frac{\lambda}{2}(\mathrm{tr}\mathbf{E})^2 + \mu\mathrm{tr}(\mathbf{E}^2) \tag{4.84}$$

is usually formulated in terms of the Green-Lagrange strain tensor. The parameter λ is called Lame's first parameter, while μ denotes the shear modulus (or Lame's second parameter). The Saint-Venant Kirchhoff model is often used for real-time applications in computer graphics. It is quickly shown (see appendix A.3 for details) that this model results in the linear relationship

$$\mathbf{S} = \frac{\partial \Psi}{\partial \mathbf{E}} = \lambda(\mathrm{tr}\mathbf{E})\mathbf{I} + 2\mu\mathbf{E} \tag{4.85}$$

between $\mathbf{S}$ and $\mathbf{E}$. Although the model can be very well suited for many large displacement problems, its formulation has several disadvantages.

It is not based on a decomposition of the strain energy function into an isochoric and volumetric part (the third invariant J is not even explicitly used). It is also not monotonic in compression and can thus break down for large compressive strains. Consequently it does not satisfy the polyconvexity condition.

4.2.3. Visco-elasticity

The stress response of a biological soft tissue does not only depend on the instantaneous strain, but also on the deformation history. This can be observed during a simple indentation experiment. The material response during the loading phase is different from the unloading (*recovery*) phase. In particular, the stress will only gradually decrease over time after the indenter has been completely removed. This relaxation process cannot be captured by purely hyperelastic models. A general approach to model this viscoelastic behavior is to express the time-dependent strain-energy function

$$\hat{\Psi} = \int_0^T G(t-s)\frac{\partial \Psi}{\partial s} ds \tag{4.86}$$

in terms of a convolution integral between the stress power and a relaxation function $G(t, \mathbf{C})$ [TCC+08]. In order to facilitate an efficient computation, it is often assumed that the relaxation function does not depend on the current strain. This approach to separate the purely hyperelastic material response from the viscoelastic behavior is called Quasi-Linear-Viscoelasticity (QLV) [Fun93]. A useful representation of the relaxation function $G(t)$ is given by the Prony series

$$G(t) = G_{\text{inf}} + \sum_{i=1}^{N} G_i e^{-t/\tau_i} \tag{4.87}$$

where G_{inf} is the long term modulus once the material is totally relaxed and τ_i are relaxation times. This model has a physical interpretation in form of a special spring-dashpot network that is called the generalized Maxwell model [Hol00]: A spring with the stiffness G_{inf} is arranged in parallel to N Maxwell elements. Each Maxwell element in turn consists of a series of one spring and one dashpot. In practice it is often much more difficult to determine G_{inf} than the instantaneous (purely elastic) modulus G_0. By noting that

$$G(t=0) = G_0 = G_{\text{inf}} + \sum_{i=1}^{N} G_i, \tag{4.88}$$

the relaxation function can be described in the equivalent form

$$G(t) = G_0 - \sum_{i=1}^{N} G_i(1 - e^{-t/\tau_i}). \tag{4.89}$$

If the relaxation function is normalized with G_0 we obtain

$$g(t) = 1 - \sum_{i=1}^{N} g_i(1 - e^{-t/\tau_i}) \tag{4.90}$$

and can subsequently express the time dependent hyperelastic material coefficients (see e.g. eq. 4.83) by the equation

$$\hat{c}_{ij}(t) = c_{ij} g(t). \tag{4.91}$$

The QLV model is considerably more computational intensive than a pure hyperelastic model. A more efficient, but less accurate approach is to use a phenomenological viscosity formulation based on the computational model. If a linear elastic model is discretized in space using the finite element method (we will discuss this procedure in detail in the next chapter) the result is the system of ordinary differential equations (ODEs)

$$\mathbf{M}\ddot{\mathcal{U}} + \mathbf{K}\mathcal{U} = \mathbf{f}^{ext}. \tag{4.92}$$

Here, $\mathcal{U}$ is a vector of nodal displacements, $\mathbf{M}$ denotes the mass matrix, $\mathbf{K}$ is the stiffness matrix and $\mathbf{f}^{ext}$ encapsulates the external forces. The idea of the widely used Rayleigh damping is to add an artificial damping term to the above equations

$$\mathbf{M}\ddot{\mathcal{U}} + \mathbf{D}\dot{\mathcal{U}} + \mathbf{K}\mathcal{U} = \mathbf{f}^{ext}. \tag{4.93}$$

In this formulation the damping matrix $\mathbf{D}$ is constructed by the linear combination

$$\mathbf{D} = \alpha\mathbf{M} + \beta\mathbf{K} \tag{4.94}$$

with the scalar coefficients α and β that control the viscoelastic behavior.
The generalization of the Rayleigh damping scheme to hyperelastic materials is straightforward. In this case, the discrete form eq. (4.92) is not a linear system of ordinary differential equations, but a non-linear one. Thus, the time-discretization of the ODEs yields a non-linear system of equations. This is typically solved by iteratively solving linear systems (Newton-Raphson algorithm). During this procedure, Rayleigh damping can be employed within each linearization step.

4.2.4. Linear elasticity

The non-linear system solve using Newton-Raphson iterations is not only computationally expensive, but can lead to instabilities especially for dynamic problems. If the deformation of the body is small (i.e. $\|\text{Grad}\mathbf{u}\| << \mathbf{I}$) and the stress-strain relationship is linear, it is not necessary to solve the non-linear problem. Instead, a computationally efficient linear elasticity model can be used. It is important to point out that this model is often used for metals. However, soft tissue deformations are usually large and the small strain assumption is thus not justified. Also, as discussed above, the material response of soft tissue is highly non-linear. It can thus be expected (and will indeed be shown in study presented in the next section) that the linear model introduces a significant error in soft tissue simulation. However, we will see in the following chapter that linear elasticity serves as an important building block for real-time capable algorithms. Therefore, the model will be presented in this section. For a more mathematical rigorous derivation of the linear model from the presented non-linear, hyperelastic model we refer to the textbook by Ogden [Ogd97].
In the context of linear elasticity it is often more convenient to use the displacement $\mathbf{u}$ (see eq. 4.3) as the primary variable. Recalling the relationship between $\mathbf{F}$ and $\mathbf{u}$ eq. (4.5) we can derive

$$\text{Grad}\mathbf{u} = \frac{\partial u_i}{\partial X_j} = \frac{\partial u_i}{\partial x_k}\frac{\partial x_k}{\partial X_j} = (\text{grad}\mathbf{u})\mathbf{F} = \text{grad}\mathbf{u}(\text{Grad}\mathbf{u} + \mathbf{I}) \tag{4.95}$$

Thus it follows that under the small strain (linear) approximation Grad$\mathbf{u}$ and grad$\mathbf{u}$ can be used interchangeably. In other words, as the reference configuration and the deformed configuration are nearly identical, i.e. the spatial and material derivative are the nearly the same. Consequently, the already defined infinitesimal strain tensor

$$\epsilon = \frac{1}{2}(\mathrm{Grad}\mathbf{u} + (\mathrm{Grad}\mathbf{u})^T) = \frac{1}{2}(\mathrm{grad}\mathbf{u} + (\mathrm{grad}\mathbf{u})^T) \tag{4.96}$$

can be alternatively expressed through a spatial derivative. Under these approximations, the rate deformation tensor

$$\mathbf{d} = \frac{1}{2}(\mathrm{grad}\mathbf{v} + (\mathrm{grad}\mathbf{v})^T) \approx \dot{\epsilon} \tag{4.97}$$

can be regarded as the time derivative of the infinitesimal strain tensor. This leads to the important finding that in the framework of linear elasticity, $\dot{\epsilon}$ is work conjugated to the Cauchy stress tensor σ (see eq. 4.61). Under the small strain assumption the strain energy rate per unit reference volume can be approximated by the strain energy rate per unit deformed volume, i.e.

$$\dot{\Psi} = J\sigma : \dot{\epsilon} \approx \sigma : \dot{\epsilon}. \tag{4.98}$$

Through this result we can establish the material law using the hyperelastic strain energy based approach. As the purpose of the small strain approximation is to achieve a completely linear formulation, the Saint-Venant Kirchhoff model is the obvious choice. With the previous results eq. (4.85) we obtain

$$\sigma = \frac{\partial \Psi}{\partial \epsilon} = \lambda \mathrm{tr}\epsilon \mathbf{I} + 2\mu\epsilon. \tag{4.99}$$

In order to compactly state the linear elastic BVP we again define the function spaces that satisfy the boundary conditions

$$V_D(\Gamma_D, \overline{\mathbf{u}}) = \{\mathbf{u} | \mathbf{u} = \overline{\mathbf{u}} \qquad \forall \mathbf{u} \in \Gamma_D\} \tag{4.100}$$

$$V_N(\Gamma_N, \overline{\mathbf{t}}) = \{\mathbf{u} | (\sigma\mathbf{n}) = \overline{\mathbf{t}} \qquad \forall \mathbf{u} \in \Gamma_N\} \tag{4.101}$$

on the Dirichlet boundary Γ_D and on the Neumann boundary Γ_N, respectively. By using the Cauchy stress in the spatial Cauchy equation of motion eq. (4.36), we can formulate the complete, displacement-based boundary value problem for linear elasticity: Find $\mathbf{u} \in C^2(\Omega) \cap C^1(\overline{\Omega}) \cap V_D(\Gamma_D, \overline{\mathbf{u}}) \cap V_N(\Gamma_N, \overline{\mathbf{t}})$ s.t.

$$\mathrm{Div}\sigma + \rho_0 \mathbf{g} = \rho_0 \ddot{\mathbf{u}} \qquad \forall \mathbf{u} \in \Omega_0 \tag{4.102}$$

$$\epsilon = \frac{1}{2}(\mathrm{Grad}\mathbf{u} + (\mathrm{Grad}\mathbf{u})^T). \tag{4.103}$$

It is very important to point out that in linear elasticity, the boundary value problem is defined in terms of the reference configuration. However, the Cauchy stress tensor is used instead of the first Piola-Kirchhoff tensor. The physical explanation for this approximation is that the reference configuration and the deformed configuration coincide and thus the Piola transform becomes unnecessary. More mathematically speaking, there exists one linear approximation of both the first Piola-Kirchhoff and the second Piola-Kirchhof stress tensor. This linear stress tensor can be identified as the Cauchy stress tensor (see Ogden for details [Ogd97]).
By noting that $\mathbf{v} = \dot{\mathbf{x}} = \dot{\mathbf{u}}$ we can also state the balance of mechanical energy for the linear elasticity formulation:

$$\frac{\mathrm{D}}{\mathrm{Dt}} \int_{\Omega_0} \frac{1}{2} \dot{\mathbf{u}}^2 \mathrm{dV} + \int_{\Omega_0} \sigma : \dot{\epsilon} \mathrm{dV} = \int_{\partial\Omega_0} \mathbf{t} \cdot \dot{\mathbf{u}} \mathrm{d}\mathbf{A} + \int_{\Omega_0} \rho \mathbf{g} \cdot \dot{\mathbf{u}} \mathrm{dV} \tag{4.104}$$

4.3. Soft tissue modeling for liver registration

We evaluated several biomechanical liver models from the literature and a new simplified model with regards to their application to intraoperative soft tissue registration. The following section summarizes the methodical approach as well as the results from this evaluation study as published in the corresponding paper [STR+11].
Obviously, the registration accuracy depends on both the boundary conditions generated from intraoperative sensor data and the complexity and parameterization of the model. The parameterization of biological soft tissue is very difficult as the material properties greatly vary under different testing conditions (*in vitro* or *in vivo*, amount of organ perfusion and loading cycle). Thus, the liver models and their parameterizations that have been proposed in the literature vary significantly [RES10] [JSZH09] [KS05]. Naturally, the question arises how these differences and additional patient-specific variations affect the registration accuracy.

Furthermore, it is interesting to analyze if complex QLV models are really needed for soft tissue registration, or if simpler hyperelastic or even linear elastic models are sufficient. Especially with real-time applications in mind it is highly desirable to keep the computation times low.
A numerical sensitivity analysis was performed for several QLV models from the literature as well as a previously proposed linear elastic model [CMG+07]. For this purpose, a finite element (FE) model of a liver phantom was subjected to typical deformation patterns that occur during surgery by applying appropriate displacement boundary conditions. We imposed deformations caused by respiratory motion as well as deformations caused by the indentation through surgical instruments. Furthermore, the models from the literature were compared to a new simplified hyperelastic liver model that uses Rayleigh damping.
Three of the most recently published viscoelastic models were selected for the study. All models were parameterized using experiments with porcine livers. Raghunathan et al. used ex-vivo measurements in a humidified chamber [RES10], whereas Jordan et al. performed the measurements on an artificially perfused liver [JSZH09]. Kim et al developed their model from in-vivo experiments [KS05]. Jordan et al. and Raghunatan et al. use a reduced polynomial model to model the hyperelastic component, while Kim et al. parameterize the Mooney-Rivlin model. All models use a QLV approach and a Prony series representation to describe the visco-elastic behavior of the material. The parameterization for the three models are shown in Table 4.1

Table 4.1.: Parameterization of QLV models for the liver. For an explanation of the viscoelastic coefficients, please refer to eq. (4.90).

Author	Model type	C_{10}	C_{01}	C_{20}	D_1	g_1	τ_1	g_2	τ_2	g_3	τ_3
Jordan et al.	Reduced polynomial, QLV	79,2	-	257	$4.38 \cdot 10^{-4}$	0.832	0.15	-	-	-	-
Raghunathan et al.	Reduced polynomial, QLV	397.7	-	208.6	$8.38 \cdot 10^{-4}$	0.503	2.1	0.185	47.1	0.142	380
Kim et al.	Mooney-Rivlin, QLV	322.96	161.47	-	$< 10^{-5}$	0.2866	1.537	0.2022	6.09	-	-

4.3.1. Simplified liver model

Organ motion compensation has to be performed in real-time during an intervention. That is why the biomechanical model does not only have to be accurate, but also very computationally efficient. We thus seek to simplify the models obtained from the literature. In particular we do not model the viscoelastic behavior with the computational intensive QLV approach, but with numerical Rayleigh damping. The hyperelastic properties of the new simplified model are described by the neo-Hookean formulation. The simplified model is parameterized according to a reference model (we chose the model by Raghunatan et al. for the study, but it should be noted that other models can be approximated as well) by performing numerical simulations of an indentation experiment on an idealized cylindrical object (Fig. 4.4). The indentation has a maximal depth of 10 mm and is performed at speeds of 1 mm/s and 10 mm/s. No-slip boundary conditions (BCs) are prescribed on the bottom of the cylinder and pressure BCs are enforced during the simulation (Fig. 4.4). The commercial FE package Abaqus (Version 6.9-1) is used to solve a discretized FE model of the cylinder. The cylinder is discretized with hybrid quadratic hexahedral element to avoid volume locking. The complete mesh contains 3264 elements and 14921 nodes. The coefficients for the simplified model that were obtained by a parametric study are listed in Table 4.2.

Table 4.2.: Parameters of the new simplified liver model.

	Neo-Hookean material		Rayleigh damping	
New simplified liver model	C_{10}	D_1	α	β
	365	$8.38 \cdot 10^{-4}$	0	0.21

4.3.2. Numerical sensitivity analysis

A geometrically realistic surface model of the human liver was obtained from a liver phantom using a laser scanner. Subsequently, a quadratic tetrahedral FE mesh (5170 elements, 8970 nodes) is constructed using the commercial software Hypermesh (Version 10). In order to realistically model the boundary conditions, we consider two different deformation

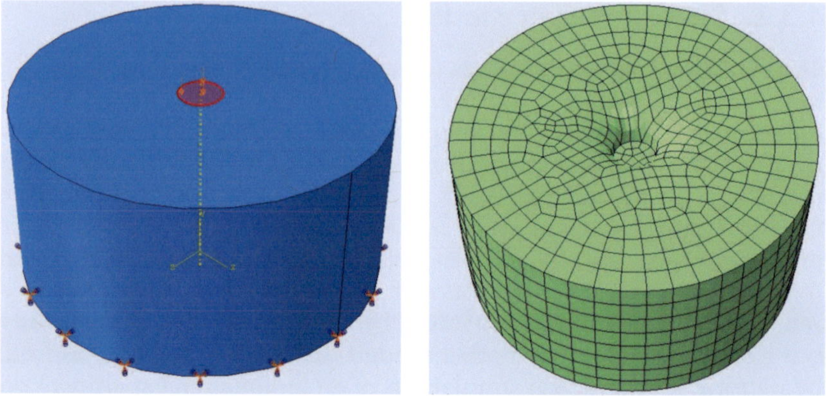

Figure 4.4.: Cylinder with boundary conditions (left), cylinder deformed by indentation (right)

patterns. The deformations caused by respiratory motion is modeled in accordance with Cash et al. [CMG+07]: The lower left side of the liver is fixed (zero displacement boundary), displacement BCs are prescribed on the upper surface of the liver (see Fig. 4.5) and all other surface remain stress-free. The maximal displacement of this deformation pattern is 48.5 mm with a mean displacement of 12.8 mm. In order to model an instrument indentation we apply local displacement boundary conditions (Fig. 4.5). The maximal displacement of the indentation is 11.07 mm with a mean displacement of 0.57 mm.
In order to assess the similarity of the registration result obtained using the different models, we compare all simulation results to a reference model. We again choose the model by Raghunathan et al. to serve as the reference model. However, it is important to point out that the choice of the reference model has only a negligible effect on the results as we are only interested in the relative differences between the models. In addition to the two other already presented QLV models and the new simplified model, we use a linear elastic model for comparison. As detailed in Table 4.3 the elastic modulus E and Poisson's ratio ν of the linear model are chosen to match the coefficients of the neo-Hookean model. All simulations are using the Abaqus FE package. We use hybrid quadratic tetrahedral elements to avoid volume locking, implicit time

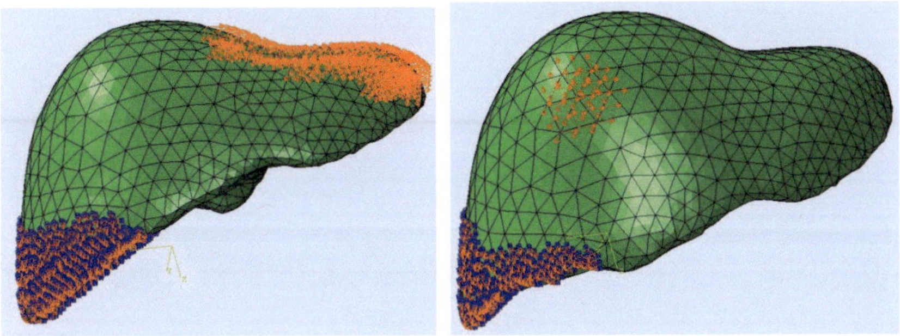

Figure 4.5.: Displacement boundary conditions (orange) to simulate organ motion caused by respiration (left) and contact with surgical instruments (right)

integration with automatic control of the increment size and a maximal half-step residual of 0.1.

Table 4.3.: Parameters of the linear elastic model

	Linear elastic material		Rayleigh damping	
Linear elastic model	Young's modulus (E)	Poisson ratio	α	β
	1987	0.36	0	0.21

In the presence of the respiratory deformation pattern all nonlinear models give nearly identical results. The maximum difference between the models is less than 0.6 mm while the maximum distance between the simplified model and the reference model is even closer (0.25 mm). However, the computation results obtained using the linear model differs substantially by a maximum distance of 3.9 mm. In case of the simulated instrument indentation the results show a different picture. Here the linear model is very close to the reference solution (0.66 mm). The simplified model also stays close to the reference (maximal distance 0.27 mm). In contrast, there is a noticeable difference of 1.1 mm between the different non-linear models.

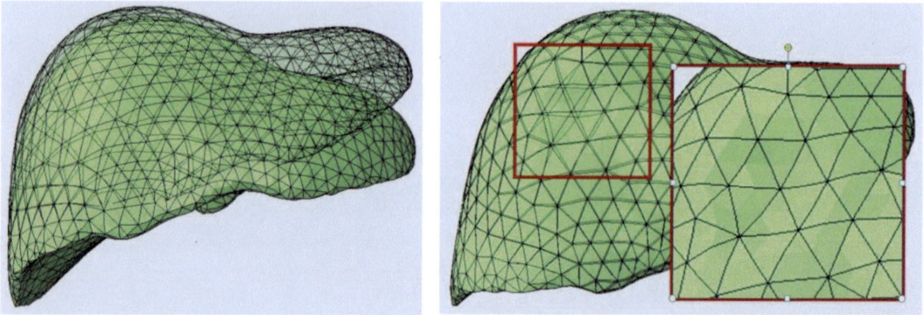

Figure 4.6.: Liver model deformed by a respiratory motion pattern (left) and by a simulated contact with surgical instruments (right)

Table 4.4.: Registration errors in comparison to a QLV reference model

	Deformations caused by surgical instruments		Deformations caused by respiratory motion	
	Maximal distance [mm]	Mean distance [mm]	Maximal distance [mm]	Mean distance [mm]
Jordan et al.	1.14	0.22	0.58	0.16
Kim et al.	1.11	0.18	0.55	0.13
Simplified model	0.27	0.007	0.25	0.07
Linear model	0.66	0.007	3.88	1.28

4.3.3. Towards real-time simulation

It can be seen that the simplified model leads to results that are very close to the QLV reference model in both scenarios. It can thus be concluded that the viscoelastic behavior can be described using the computationally efficient Rayleigh damping. It can also be observed that the linear model is very inaccurate in the first scenario. This can be attributed to the large rotational component of the deformation pattern that cannot be adequately captured by the linear Cauchy deformation tensor. It is interesting to note that these results are in line with the results obtained by Cash et al. using linear modeling (max. displacement of 3-4 cm and error around 4 mm). Due to the rotation-invariance of the non-linear Cauchy-Green deformation tensor, all geometrically non-linear models lead to very similar deformation fields. Interestingly, the

model complexity and parameterization have only negligible effects. This behavior has previously been observed for the brain shift problem in neurosurgery [HWM06].
In the instrument indentation setting, the linear model performs much better. Its distance to the reference model is roughly twice as large (0.66 mm) as the distance of the neo-Hookean model (0.27 mm). This can be attributed to the comparatively small overall deformations and in particular to the absence of large rotational components in the deformation pattern. It is important to note that the parameterization of the model plays a bigger role than in the previous scenario. However, even though the stiffness parameters of the models vary considerably, all models perform reasonably well (max. distance 1.14 mm).
The different parameterization of the models form the literature can largely be attributed to the different testing conditions. These differences are large if compared to patient-specific variations. Thus, the results of the study suggest that a difficult patient-specific parameterization of the model might not be necessary for intraoperative soft tissue registration. It is important to note that these findings are only true for displacement-zero traction boundary conditions. As explained in the previous chapter, this type of BCs naturally arises from intraoperative imaging modalities (e.g. endoscopes, ultrasound). However, if surface tractions were to be prescribed on the liver surface (e.g. by using an intraoperative force sensor) the sensitivity of the registration accuracy with regards to the model parameterization would be much higher.
It can be concluded that linear models are not suitable for liver registration. Due to the large deformations, a rotation-invariant, geometrically non-linear formulation has to be employed. It was also demonstrated that simple Rayleigh damping can be used instead of complex QLV models without sacrificing accuracy.
The next chapter will be dedicated to exploring fast finite element solving techniques for biomechanically based soft tissue registration. Building on the primary result of the presented study - that soft tissue registration requires the use of a geometrically non-linear model, but that the material law is not very important - it will be shown how so called corotated elements are can lead to an efficient, yet accurate model for real-time registration.

A computer will do what you tell it to do, but that may be much different from what you had in mind.
— Joseph Weizenbaum

5. Real-time finite element formulation

In this chapter, a computational soft tissue model for the non-rigid registration process is developed. We start by outlining a variational form of the BVP for linear elasticity. Subsequently it is shown how the variational form can be discretized in space using the finite element (FE) method and how to obtain the fully time-discrete formulation using time integration techniques. With respect to a future real-time application of the approach, a FE model based on quadratic corotated tetrahedra that is very accurate and efficient is presented. The accuracy of the model is demonstrated in different numerical studies. We also describe a lightweight solution for distributed computing in the context of computer assisted surgery.

5.1. Variational formulation

5.1.1. Weak solution in Sobolev spaces

The basic idea of a finite element method is to discretize the physical problem in a so called weak (or variational) form instead of its classical strong formulation. For this purpose we define the test functions $\delta\mathbf{u} \in C_0^\infty \cap V_D(\Gamma_D, 0)$ with compact support that vanish on the Dirichlet boundary Γ_D. Then, we demand that the L^2 scalar product

$$\int_{\Omega_0} (\mathrm{Div}\,\sigma + \rho_0 \mathbf{g} - \rho_0 \ddot{\mathbf{u}})\, \delta\mathbf{u}\, \mathrm{dV}_0 = 0 \qquad \forall \delta\mathbf{u} \tag{5.1}$$

between the residual of the partial differential equation (PDE) and the test functions vanishes for all $\delta\mathbf{u}$. Rephrasing the divergence term using the product differentiation rule

$$\mathrm{Div}\sigma \cdot \delta\mathbf{u} = \mathrm{Div}(\sigma\delta\mathbf{u}) - \sigma : \mathrm{Grad}\delta\mathbf{u} \tag{5.2}$$

and application of the divergence theorem yields

$$\int_{\Omega_0} \mathrm{Div}\sigma \cdot \delta\mathbf{u}\mathrm{dV}_0 = \int_{\Omega_0} \mathrm{Div}(\sigma\delta\mathbf{u})\mathrm{dV}_0 - \int_{\Omega_0} \sigma : \mathrm{Grad}\delta\mathbf{u}\mathrm{dV}_0 \tag{5.3}$$

$$= \int_{\Gamma_N} \mathbf{t} \cdot \delta\mathbf{u}\mathrm{d}\mathbf{A}_0 - \int_{\Omega_0} \sigma : \mathrm{Grad}\delta\mathbf{u}\mathrm{dV}_0. \tag{5.4}$$

Here, $\mathbf{t}$ are the prescribed traction boundary conditions on Γ_N. Inserting this in eq. 5.1 gives rise to the weak form of Cauchy's equation of motion:

$$\int_{\Omega_0} \sigma : \mathrm{Grad}\delta\mathbf{u}\mathrm{dV}_0 - \int_{\Gamma_N} \mathbf{t} \cdot \delta\mathbf{u}\mathrm{d}\mathbf{A}_0 - \int_{\Omega_0} (\rho_0\mathbf{g} \cdot \delta\mathbf{u} + \rho_0\ddot{\mathbf{u}} \cdot \delta\mathbf{u})\,\mathrm{dV}_0 = 0. \tag{5.5}$$

It is apparent, that each $\mathbf{u}$ which solves the original boundary value problem (BVP) is also a solution to the weak formulation. It can also be shown that each $\mathbf{u} \in C^2(\Omega) \cap C^1(\overline{\Omega}) \cap V_D(\Gamma_D,\overline{\mathbf{u}}) \cap V_N(\Gamma_N,\overline{\mathbf{t}})$ for which eq. (5.5) holds is also a solution of the classical PDE [Bra07]. However, if we only assume $\mathbf{u} \in V_D(\Gamma_D,\overline{\mathbf{u}}) \cap V_N(\Gamma_N,\overline{\mathbf{t}})$ and not $\mathbf{u} \in C^2(\Omega) \cap C^1(\overline{\Omega})$, then the weak formulation has more solutions than the classical one. Through the definition of weak derivatives the space of all solutions $\mathbf{u} \in V_D(\Gamma_D,\overline{\mathbf{u}}) \cap V_N(\Gamma_N,\overline{\mathbf{t}})$ to eq. 5.5 can be identified with the Sobolev space $H^1(\Omega)$ [Bra07]. It should be noted that there are physical problems (e.g. shock problems) which have no classical solutions, but do have a solution in $H^1(\Omega)$.

The solution space is not only a Sobolev space, but also a Hilbert space (hence the notation $H^1(\Omega)$). Thus, the powerful tools of functional analysis open up a natural way of discretizing the weak form by finite element based techniques. Also, the concept of weak solutions in Sobolev spaces is a very useful tool in the analysis of uniqueness and existence of solutions to BVP. In particular, the Lax-Milgram theorem establishes that the bilinear form (5.1) has a unique solution if it is strongly coercive [Bra07].

5.1.2. Static formulation: Minimizing energy functionals

In the following section we will formulate the static problem in terms of minimizing the total energy of $\mathcal{B}$. It will become apparent that this variational formulation is identical to the weak formulation. This physics-based derivation provides an elegant and intuitive access to weak formulations and will be extensively used in this thesis.
The total potential energy of the system can be formally derived from the balance of mechanical energy for linear elasticity eq. (4.104). For this purpose we assume that each particle in $\mathcal{B}$ is at rest at the beginning of the simulation, i.e. $\mathbf{v}(\mathbf{x}, t = 0) = 0$. Omitting the inertia forces (static approximation) and integrating eq. (4.104) over time then yields

$$\Pi(\mathbf{u}) = \int_{\Omega_0} \sigma : \epsilon \mathrm{dV}_0 - \int_{\partial\Omega_0} \mathbf{t} \cdot \mathbf{u} \mathrm{d}\mathbf{A}_0 - \int_{\Omega_0} \rho \mathbf{g} \cdot \mathbf{u} \mathrm{dV}_0. \tag{5.6}$$

The solution to the static problem can be interpreted as the configuration that minimizes this energy functional. The principle of stationary potential energy states a necessary condition for a stationary point in $\Pi(\mathbf{u})$: It requires the directional derivative with respect to the displacements $\mathbf{u}$

$$\Pi(\mathbf{u}, \delta\mathbf{u}) = D_{\delta\mathbf{u}}\Pi(\mathbf{u}) = \frac{\mathrm{d}}{\mathrm{dh}}\Pi(\mathbf{u} + h\delta\mathbf{u})\bigg|_{h=0} = 0 \tag{5.7}$$

to vanish in all directions [Hol00]. Carrying out the variation on the internal elastic energy yields:

$$D_{\delta\mathbf{u}}\Pi(\mathbf{u})_{int} = \frac{\mathrm{d}}{\mathrm{dh}} \int_{\Omega_0} \sigma : \epsilon \mathrm{dV}_0 \bigg|_{h=0} \tag{5.8}$$

$$= \frac{\mathrm{d}}{\mathrm{dh}} \int_{\Omega_0} \sigma : \frac{1}{2}((\nabla\mathbf{u} + h\nabla\delta\mathbf{u}) + (\nabla\mathbf{u} + h\nabla\delta\mathbf{u})^T)\mathrm{dV}_0 \bigg|_{h=0} \tag{5.9}$$

$$= \int_{\Omega_0} \sigma : \frac{1}{2}(\delta\nabla\mathbf{u} + \delta\nabla\mathbf{u}^T)\mathrm{dV}_0 \bigg|_{h=0} \tag{5.10}$$

$$= \int_{\Omega_0} \sigma : \delta\frac{1}{2}(\nabla\mathbf{u} + \nabla\mathbf{u}^T)\mathrm{dV}_0 = \int_{\Omega_0} \sigma : \delta\epsilon \mathrm{dV}_0 \tag{5.11}$$

Similarly, the external energies (loads) can be expressed as

$$D_{\delta\mathbf{u}}\Pi(\mathbf{u})_{ext} = \frac{\mathrm{d}}{\mathrm{dh}}\int_{\partial\Omega_0}\mathbf{t}\cdot(\mathbf{u}+h\delta\mathbf{u})\mathrm{dA}_0 + \frac{\mathrm{d}}{\mathrm{dh}}\int_{\Omega_0}\rho\mathbf{g}\cdot(\mathbf{u}+h\delta\mathbf{u})\mathrm{dV}_0\bigg|_{h=0} \tag{5.12}$$

$$= \int_{\partial\Omega_0}\mathbf{t}\cdot\delta\mathbf{u}\mathrm{dA}_0 + \int_{\Omega_0}\rho\mathbf{g}\cdot\delta\mathbf{u}\mathrm{dV}_0 \tag{5.13}$$

and thus the complete variational form is

$$D_{\delta\mathbf{u}}\Pi(\mathbf{u}) = D_{\delta\mathbf{u}}\Pi(\mathbf{u})_{int} + D_{\delta\mathbf{u}}\Pi(\mathbf{u})_{ext} = 0 \tag{5.14}$$

$$\Leftrightarrow \quad \int_{\Omega_0}\sigma : \delta\epsilon\mathrm{dV}_0 = \int_{\partial\Omega_0}\mathbf{t}\cdot\delta\mathbf{u}\mathrm{dA}_0 + \int_{\Omega_0}\rho\mathbf{g}\cdot\delta\mathbf{u}\mathrm{dV}_0. \tag{5.15}$$

We can thus summarize the variational formulation of the static elasticity problem: Find the displacement field $\mathbf{u} \in V = H^1(\Omega) \cap V_D(\Gamma_D, \bar{\mathbf{u}}) \cap V_N(\Gamma_N, \bar{\mathbf{t}})$, s.t. eq. (5.15) holds for all $\delta\mathbf{u} \in H^1 \cap V_D(\Gamma_D, 0)$. It can be quickly shown (symmetry of σ) that the variational form is equivalent to the weak formulation.

5.1.3. Dynamic formulation: Hamiltonian variational principle

In the dynamic case, the intuitive formulation in terms of minimizing the elastic energy is replaced by the principle of least action [Ibr09]. More formally we now seek the stationary point of the Hamiltonian variational principle.
With the same assumptions that we made in the static case, we can derive the Lagrangian

$$L(\mathbf{u}) = \Pi(\mathbf{u}) - \mathcal{K}(\dot{\mathbf{u}}) \tag{5.16}$$

$$= \int_{\Omega_0}\sigma : \epsilon\mathrm{dV}_0 - \int_{\partial\Omega_0}\mathbf{t}\cdot\mathbf{u}\mathrm{d}\mathbf{A}_0 - \int_{\Omega_0}\rho\mathbf{g}\cdot\mathbf{u}\mathrm{dV}_0 - \int_{\Omega_0}\frac{1}{2}\rho_0\dot{\mathbf{u}}^2\mathrm{dV}_0 \tag{5.17}$$

of the system [HG01]. The solution to the dynamic elasticity problem can then be regarded as a stationary point of the Hamiltonian variational principle

$$D_{\delta\mathbf{u}}H(\mathbf{u}) = \int_0^T L(\mathbf{u})\mathrm{dt} \tag{5.18}$$

We compute the variation of the kinetic part of the Hamiltonian using integration by parts:

$$D_{\delta\mathbf{u}}H_{kin}(\mathbf{u}) = \frac{\mathrm{d}}{\mathrm{dh}}\int_0^T -\int_{\Omega_0}\frac{1}{2}\rho_0(\frac{\mathrm{d}(\mathbf{u}+h\delta\mathbf{u})}{\mathrm{dt}})^2\mathrm{dV_0dt}\bigg|_{h=0} \tag{5.19}$$

$$= -\int_{\Omega_0}\int_0^T \frac{1}{2}\rho_0 2\frac{\mathrm{d}(\mathbf{u}+h\delta\mathbf{u})}{\mathrm{dt}}\frac{\mathrm{d}}{\mathrm{dh}}\frac{\mathrm{d}(\mathbf{u}+h\delta\mathbf{u})}{\mathrm{dt}}\mathrm{dtdV_0}\bigg|_{h=0} \tag{5.20}$$

$$= \int_{\Omega_0}\left(-\left[\rho_0\frac{\mathrm{d}(\mathbf{u}+h\delta\mathbf{u})}{\mathrm{dt}}\delta\mathbf{u}\right]_0^T + \int_0^T \rho_0\frac{\mathrm{d}^2(\mathbf{u}+h\delta\mathbf{u})}{\mathrm{dt}^2}\delta\mathbf{u}\mathrm{dt}\right)\mathrm{dV_0}\bigg|_{h=0} \tag{5.21}$$

$$= \int_{\Omega_0}\left(-\rho_0\frac{\mathrm{d}\mathbf{u}}{\mathrm{dt}}\underbrace{\delta\mathbf{u}(T)}_{=0}+\rho_0\frac{\mathrm{d}\mathbf{u}}{\mathrm{dt}}\underbrace{\delta\mathbf{u}(0)}_{=0}+\int_0^T\rho_0\frac{\mathrm{d}^2\mathbf{u}}{\mathrm{dt}^2}\delta\mathbf{u}\mathrm{dt}\right)\mathrm{dV_0} \tag{5.22}$$

$$= \int_0^T\int_{\Omega_0}\rho_0\ddot{\mathbf{u}}\delta\mathbf{u}\mathrm{dV_0dt} \tag{5.23}$$

The final result was obtained by imposing that the variations are zero at both limits of the time interval. By using the previous results obtained in the static case eq. (5.15), the complete variation of the Hamiltonian reads

$$D_{\delta\mathbf{u}}H(\mathbf{u}) = \tag{5.24}$$

$$\int_0^T\left(\int_{\Omega_0}\rho_0\ddot{\mathbf{u}}\delta\mathbf{u}\mathrm{dV_0} + \sigma:\delta\epsilon\mathrm{dV_0} - \int_{\partial\Omega_0}\mathbf{t}\cdot\delta\mathbf{u}\mathrm{dA_0} - \int_{\Omega_0}\rho\mathbf{g}\cdot\delta\mathbf{u}\mathrm{dV_0}\right)\mathrm{dt}. \tag{5.25}$$

It is reasonable to require the above equation to hold for all T during the simulation. Thus, the dynamic problem can be posed in its corresponding time-differential, space variational form: Find the displacement field $\mathbf{u} \in V = H^1(\Omega) \cap V_D(\Gamma_D,\overline{\mathbf{u}}) \cap V_N(\Gamma_N,\overline{\mathbf{t}})$, s.t.

$$\int_{\Omega_0} \rho_0 \ddot{\mathbf{u}} \delta \mathbf{u} \mathrm{dV}_0 + \int_{\Omega_0} \boldsymbol{\sigma} : \delta \boldsymbol{\epsilon} \mathrm{dV}_0 - \int_{\partial\Omega_0} \mathbf{t} \cdot \delta \mathbf{u} \mathrm{dA}_0 - \int_{\Omega_0} \rho \mathbf{g} \cdot \delta \mathbf{u} \mathrm{dV}_0 = 0 \tag{5.26}$$

holds for all $\delta\mathbf{u} \in H^1 \cap V_D(\Gamma_D,0)$.

5.2. Finite element discretization

The idea of the finite element discretization technique is to not look for a solution $\mathbf{u}$ to the variational problem in the infinite-dimensional space V of continuous functions, but to an approximated solution $\mathbf{u}_h$ in a suitable finite-dimensional, discrete sub-space $V_h \subset V$. This subspace is typically spanned by piecewise continuous polynomial functions that have *small* support. In order to define these function spaces, Ω is divided into different polyhedral elements (Fig. 5.1). In this context the boundary of Ω is required to be sufficiently smoothed which is formalized through the assumption that Ω is a Lipschitz domain.

When constructing the finite element space we are facing the fundamental problem that is associated with every discretization technique: How to find the best approximation to the correct solution with a given amount of complexity in terms of degrees of freedom of the discrete system. An important reason for the success of the FE-method are the powerful and elegant tools that are available for a-priori error approximation. At the core, Céa's lemma states that the finite element approximation $\mathbf{u}_h$ is the near best fit to the solution $\mathbf{u}$ in the norm associated with H^1 [Bra07]. Geometrically speaking, the discrete solution $\mathbf{u}_h$ is the orthogonal projection of $\mathbf{u}$ into V_h with respect to the inner product that is induced by the bilinear form (5.1). It follows that the construction of the subspace V_h is crucial for the accuracy of the method.

The convergence of FE methods is typically studied in suitable mesh-dependent norms. Thus, several a-priori error estimates exist for different norms and different finite element types. For finite element spaces that are spanned by piecewise polynomials of order p on tetrahedral and hexahedral elements, it can be shown that the convergence rate for is of order $p+1$ if the real solution is sufficiently smooth. However, the latter

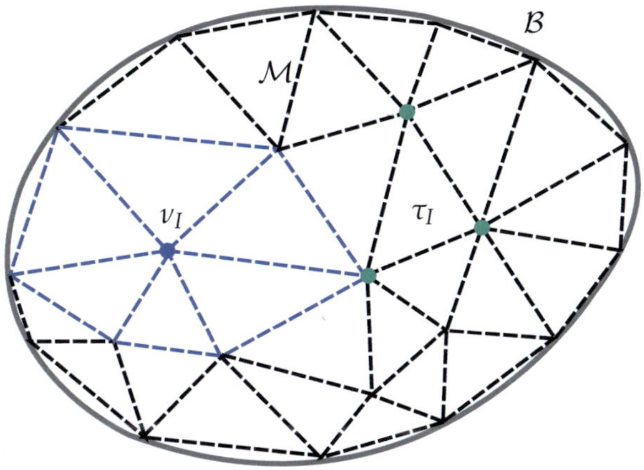

Figure 5.1.: A two dimensional body $\mathcal{B}$ (grey line) is discretized with a triangular finite element mesh $\mathcal{M}$ (dashed lines). The set of vertices $\mathcal{V}_I$ that form the element τ_I is shown in green, while the set of all elements $\mathcal{E}_I$ around the vertex ν_I is colored blue.

is usually not the case in many applications. Thus first or second order polynomials are typically used for elasticity problems.
A finite element mesh $\mathcal{M}$ with elements τ_I and n vertices ν_I is defined to support the basis functions that span the solution space V_h. We denote the set of all elements τ_J around the vertex ν_I with $\mathcal{E}_I$. Similarly $\mathcal{V}_I$ is the set of vertices that form the element τ_I. Typically so called nodal basis functions N_J are used. Each nodal functions N_J satisfies

$$N_J(\nu_I) = \delta_{IJ} \tag{5.27}$$

i.e. it is zero at every other node except the associated J-th node (δ-property). Furthermore, the nodal basis function satisfy the *partition of unity*

$$\sum_{J \in \mathcal{V}_I} N_J(\mathbf{x}) = 1 \quad \forall \mathbf{x} \in \tau_I \tag{5.28}$$

and have a *small*, compact support, i.e.

$$N_J(\mathbf{x}) = 0 \quad \forall \mathbf{x} \notin \mathcal{E}_J. \tag{5.29}$$

The nodal basis functions for linear and quadratic tetrahedral elements can be found in appendix A.4. In order to discretize the weak formulation, $\mathbf{u}_h$ is expressed by the linear combination

$$\mathbf{u}_h(t) = \mathbf{u}_h = \sum_{J=1}^{n} \mathcal{U}_J N_J = \mathcal{U}_J N_J = \mathcal{U}_{jJ} N_{jJ} \tag{5.30}$$

of the n basis functions N_J with the time dependent coefficients $\mathcal{U}$ or $\mathcal{U}(t)$ (in the above equation and from here on out summation over repeated indices is implied). As a direct consequence of the δ-property, the coefficients $\mathcal{U}(t)$ coincide with the displacements of the element nodes when using nodal basis functions. Due to the special form of the basis functions, the solution $\mathbf{u}_h$ is C^0-continuous and we have $V_h \subset V$. It is only through this so called conformal finite element space that statements on uniqueness and existence of solutions can be directly transferred from the continuous to the discrete problem.
For later use, we also introduce the displacement gradient

$$\nabla \mathbf{u} = \nabla(\mathcal{U}_J N_J) = \mathcal{U}_J \nabla N_J. \tag{5.31}$$

It is theoretically possible to use different function spaces for $\mathbf{u}_h$ and the test functions $\delta \mathbf{u}_h$. However, in practice we usually choose these spaces to be the same (Galerkin method). Thus we have

$$\delta \mathbf{u} = \sum_{I=1}^{n} \delta \mathcal{U}_I N_I = \delta \mathcal{U}_I N_I \tag{5.32}$$

5.2.1. Matrix formulation

By inserting the basis functions and the test functions into the variational formulation (5.26) and performing numerical integration, a linear system of ordinary differential equations can be derived. In the following we sketch this procedure and derive the load vector as well as the mass and the stiffness matrix.

We start by inserting the test functions into the expression for the external forces eq. (5.13) to derive

$$D_{\delta\mathcal{U}}\Pi(\mathbf{u}_h)_{ext} = \int_{\partial\Omega_0} \mathbf{t}\cdot(\delta\mathcal{U}_I N_I)\,\mathrm{dA}_0 + \int_{\Omega_0} \rho g\cdot(\delta\mathcal{U}_I N_I)\,\mathrm{dV}_0 \tag{5.33}$$

$$= \delta\mathcal{U}_I\left(\int_{\partial\Omega_0} \mathbf{t}\cdot N_I \mathrm{dA}_0 + \int_{\Omega_0} \rho g\cdot N_I \mathrm{dV}_0\right) = \delta\mathcal{U}_I \mathbf{f}_I^{ext}. \tag{5.34}$$

As the test functions are polynomials, the surface and volume integrals in (5.34) can be accurately and efficiently evaluated using numerical integration techniques such as Gaussian quadrature. For an overview on this topic we refer to Zienkiewicz et al. [ZT77]. The resulting external load vector $\mathbf{f}_I^{ext}$ (sometimes also written as $\mathbf{f}^{ext}$ or f_{iI}^{ext}) denotes the force that acts on each node P_I in the spatial direction j. Its length is thus $3n$.
Similarly, the discretization of the inertia forces (variation of kinetic energy) (5.23) yields

$$D_{\delta\mathcal{U}}\Pi(\mathbf{u}_h)_{kin} = \int_{\Omega_0} \rho\,(\ddot{\mathcal{U}}_J N_J)\,(\delta\mathcal{U}_I N_I)\,\mathrm{dV}_0 = \delta\mathcal{U}_I \int_{\Omega_0} \rho N_J \ddot{\mathcal{U}}_J N_I \mathrm{dV}_0 \tag{5.35}$$

$$= \delta\mathcal{U}_I\left(\int_{\Omega_0} \rho N_J N_I \mathrm{dV}_0\right)\ddot{\mathcal{U}}_J = \delta\mathcal{U}_I \mathbf{M}_{IJ}\ddot{\mathcal{U}}_J. \tag{5.36}$$

The entries of the so called mass matrix $\mathbf{M}_{IJ}$ (sometimes also denoted with $\mathbf{M}$ or $\mathbf{M}_{iIjJ}$) are again computed using numerical integration. The vector $\ddot{\mathcal{U}}_J$ (or simply $\ddot{\mathcal{U}}$) is the vector of nodal accelerations.
The internal forces obviously depend on the deformation field $\mathbf{u}_h$ and thus on the vector of nodal displacement $\mathcal{U}$ (i.e. the coefficients of the basis functions). If the displacement is known we can compute the internal nodal forces using numerical integration. Due to the symmetry of σ we can derive:

$$D_{\delta\mathcal{U}}\Pi(\mathbf{u}_h)_{int} = \int_{\Omega_0} \sigma : \delta\epsilon \mathrm{dV}_0 = \int_{\Omega_0} \sigma : \frac{1}{2}\left(\delta\nabla\mathbf{u} + (\delta\nabla\mathbf{u})^T\right)\mathrm{dV}_0 \tag{5.37}$$

$$= \int_{\Omega_0} \sigma : \delta\nabla\mathbf{u}\mathrm{dV}_0 = \int_{\Omega_0} \sigma : (\delta\mathcal{U}_I \nabla N_I)\,\mathrm{dV}_0 \tag{5.38}$$

$$= \delta\mathcal{U}_{iI}\int_{\Omega_0} \sigma_{ik}(\nabla N)_{kI}\mathrm{dV}_0 = \delta\mathcal{U}_{iI}\int_{\Omega_0} \hat{f}_{iI}^{X,int}\mathrm{dV}_0 \tag{5.39}$$

$$= \delta\mathcal{U}_{iI} f_{iI}^{int} = \delta\mathcal{U}_I \mathbf{f}_I^{int} \tag{5.40}$$

Here, $\hat{f}_{iI}^{X,int}$ denotes internal force density. For implicit integration schemes or non-linear static solvers of Newton-Raphson type, the tangent stiffness matrix

$$\mathbf{K}_{IJ} = K_{iIjJ} = \frac{\partial f_{iI}^{int}}{\partial \mathcal{U}_{jJ}} = \int_{\Omega_0} \frac{\partial \hat{f}_{iI}^{X,int}}{\partial \mathcal{U}_{jJ}} \mathrm{dV}_0 = \sum_{\tau} \int_{\tau} \frac{\partial \hat{f}_{iI}^{X,int}}{\partial \mathcal{U}_{jJ}} \mathrm{dV}_0 = \sum_{\tau} \mathbf{K}^{\tau} \quad (5.41)$$

is necessary. From the above equation it is apparent how the global stiffness matrix $\mathbf{K}_{IJ}$ is constructed: First, the integrals in the above equation are evaluated on a per-element basis. Due to the small support of the basis functions, only few integrals (e.g. 12 for the linear tetrahedron) have to be evaluated for each row. These elemental matrices $\mathbf{K}^{\tau}$ are then added into the global data structure (*matrix assembly*).
For the linear elastic model, the entries of the tangent stiffness matrix can be computed as (please refer to the appendix A.5 for details):

$$K_{iIjJ} = \int_{\Omega_0} \left(\mu \nabla N_{iJ} \nabla N_{jI} + \mu \delta_{IJ} \sum_{l=1}^{3} \nabla N_{il} \nabla N_{jl} + \lambda \nabla N_{iI} \nabla N_{jJ} \right) \mathrm{dV}_0 \quad (5.42)$$

Here, δ_{IJ} again denotes the Kronecker-delta symbol and μ, λ are the material parameters. For linear elasticity, there is

$$\mathbf{f}^{int} = \mathbf{K}_{IJ} \mathcal{U}_J. \quad (5.43)$$

The global matrices $\mathbf{M}, \mathbf{K}$ are symmetric, positive definite sparse matrices. Their sparsity pattern depends on the mesh topology and is thus is irregular for unstructured grids.
Using the obtained discretization of the external, inertia and internal forces we can state the discrete variational form

$$D_{\delta \mathbf{u}} \Pi(\mathbf{u})_{kin} + D_{\delta \mathbf{u}} \Pi(\mathbf{u})_{int} = D_{\delta \mathbf{u}} \Pi(\mathbf{u})_{ext} \quad (5.44)$$

$$\Leftrightarrow \quad \delta \mathcal{U}_I \mathbf{M}_{IJ} \ddot{\mathcal{U}}_J + \delta \mathcal{U}_I \mathbf{f}^{int} = \delta \mathcal{U}_I \mathbf{f}_I^{ext} \quad (5.45)$$

As the equation holds for all variations $\delta \mathcal{U}_I$, the variational form can be stated as a system of second order ordinary differential equations (ODE):

$$\mathbf{M} \ddot{\mathcal{U}} + \mathbf{f}^{int} = \mathbf{f}^{ext} \quad (5.46)$$

This equality also holds for non-linear problems. For the linear elastic formulation, the internal nodal forces depend linearly on the nodal displacements eq. (5.43) and we can express the equilibrium equations through the following system of linear second order ODE's:

$$\mathbf{M}\ddot{\mathcal{U}} + \mathbf{K}\mathcal{U} = \mathbf{f}^{ext} \tag{5.47}$$

Neumann boundary conditions (forces on the surface) are reflected in the formulation through the external forces $\mathbf{f}^{ext}$. In the following section, we will see how Dirichlet boundary conditions (prescribed displacements) can be imposed during the linear system solve once the system of ODEs has been discretized using time integration techniques.

5.3. Time integration

In this section we derive the full discretization, i.e. we discretize the ODEs in time to derive a linear system of equations. The methods are presented with linear elasticity in mind, but easily generalize to non-linear problems.

For viscoelastic models the internal nodal forces also encapsulate the viscoelastic behavior (see section 4.2.3). Consequently, we can define the tangent damping matrix

$$\mathbf{D}_{IJ} = D_{iIjJ} = \frac{\partial f_{iI}^{int}}{\partial \dot{\mathcal{U}}_{jJ}} \tag{5.48}$$

in addition to the tangent stiffness matrix eq. (5.43). Time integration methods can be categorized into explicit and implicit methods. The explicit methods enforce the equilibrium (5.46) only at the beginning of the time step at the current time t, whereas implicit algorithms enforce it at the end of the time step at time $t + \Delta t$ (Δt is the time step size). Explicit methods are very computationally efficient, as their computation only require matrix-vector operations. In contrast, implicit methods require solving a system of equations for every time step. However, explicit methods are only conditionally stable. Especially for stiff systems, they need very small timesteps to remain stable. Thus they are often a poor choice for soft tissue simulations especially for nearly incompressible material models [SM03]. For real-time deformable model problems, implicit

methods have emerged as the dominant means for time discretization [BW98].
In the following, we describe the dynamic equilibrium (5.46) at time $t+\Delta t$ under the assumption that the system is in equilibrium at time t. From now on we denote the point in time for each nodal quantity with left superscript (e.g. $t+\Delta t$). The superscript t which indicates the current time is omitted when apparent from the context. We also define

$$\mathrm{d}\mathcal{U} = {}^{t+\Delta t}\mathcal{U} - {}^{t}\mathcal{U} \qquad \text{and} \qquad \mathrm{d}\dot{\mathcal{U}} = {}^{t+\Delta t}\dot{\mathcal{U}} - {}^{t}\dot{\mathcal{U}}. \tag{5.49}$$

Using the tangent stiffness matrix and the tangent damping matrix, we can express the first order Taylor expansion of $\mathbf{f}^{int}$ around t as

$$\begin{aligned} {}^{t+\Delta t}\mathbf{f}^{int} &= {}^{t}\mathbf{f}^{int} + \frac{\partial \mathbf{f}^{int}}{\partial \dot{\mathcal{U}}}({}^{t+\Delta t}\dot{\mathcal{U}} - {}^{t}\dot{\mathcal{U}}) + \frac{\partial \mathbf{f}^{int}}{\partial \mathcal{U}}({}^{t+\Delta t}\mathcal{U} - {}^{t}\mathcal{U}) && (5.50)\\ &= {}^{t}\mathbf{f}^{int} + \mathbf{D}\mathrm{d}\dot{\mathcal{U}} + \mathbf{K}\mathrm{d}\mathcal{U}. && (5.51)\end{aligned}$$

As the external forces (*dead loads*) do not depend on the deformation, i.e.

$${}^{t+\Delta t}\mathbf{f}^{ext} = {}^{t}\mathbf{f}^{ext}, \tag{5.52}$$

the equilibrium at time $t+\Delta t$ is

$$\mathbf{M}\ddot{\mathcal{U}} + \mathbf{D}\mathrm{d}\dot{\mathcal{U}} + \mathbf{K}\mathrm{d}\mathcal{U} = \mathbf{f}^{ext} - \mathbf{f}^{int}. \tag{5.53}$$

In the static, non-linear case the above equation reduces to a Newton-Raphson iteration algorithm. It is solved by first calculating $\mathbf{D},\mathbf{K}$ for $\mathcal{U}$, then solving eq. 5.53 for $\mathrm{d}\mathcal{U}$ and finally performing the update $\mathcal{U} = \mathcal{U} + \mathrm{d}\mathcal{U}$. This procedure is typically repeated until $\mathrm{d}\mathcal{U}$ is below a certain threshold.

5.3.1. Implicit Euler method

The implicit Euler scheme is unconditionally stable and emerged as the de-facto standard for real-time deformable model simulation. However, it has only a convergence order of one. The update equations for the implicit Euler time integration technique are:

$$\begin{aligned} {}^{t+\Delta t}\dot{\mathcal{U}} &= {}^{t}\dot{\mathcal{U}} + h({}^{t+\Delta t}\ddot{\mathcal{U}})\\ {}^{t+\Delta t}\mathcal{U} &= {}^{t}\mathcal{U} + h({}^{t+\Delta t}\dot{\mathcal{U}}) \end{aligned} \tag{5.54}$$

Upon inserting these update equations into the equilibrium condition eq. (5.53) we obtain the linear system

$$\mathbf{A}\mathrm{d}\dot{\mathcal{U}} = \mathbf{b} \tag{5.55}$$

with the system matrix

$$\mathbf{A} = \mathbf{M} + \Delta t\mathbf{D} + \Delta t^2\mathbf{K} \tag{5.56}$$

and the effective load

$$\mathbf{b} = \mathbf{f}^{ext} - \mathbf{f}^{int} - \Delta t^2\mathbf{K}\dot{\mathcal{U}}. \tag{5.57}$$

Thus, for each time step one linear system of equations has to be solved. Once the system solve has been performed, the new velocities, displacements and accelerations can be obtained through the update equations (5.54).

5.3.2. Newmark method

In some cases it is desirable to achieve a higher accuracy for the time discretization technique. An attractive alternative is offered by the constant-average-acceleration scheme of the β-Newmark method [BLM00]. It's additional computational overhead is negligible compared to the implicit Euler scheme and it is of second order accuracy. The update equations are:

$$\begin{aligned} {}^{t+\Delta t}\ddot{\mathcal{U}} &= \frac{4}{\Delta t^2}\left({}^{t+\Delta t}\mathrm{d}\mathcal{U}\right) - \frac{4}{\Delta t}\,{}^{t}\dot{\mathcal{U}} - {}^{t}\ddot{\mathcal{U}} \\ {}^{t+\Delta t}\dot{\mathcal{U}} &= {}^{t}\dot{\mathcal{U}} + \frac{\Delta t}{2}\left({}^{t}\ddot{\mathcal{U}} + {}^{t+\Delta t}\ddot{\mathcal{U}}\right) \end{aligned} \tag{5.58}$$

By again defining a system matrix

$$\mathbf{A} = \frac{4}{\Delta t^2}\mathbf{M} + \frac{2}{\Delta t}\mathbf{D} + \mathbf{K} \tag{5.59}$$

and the effective load

$$\mathbf{b} = {}^{t}\mathbf{f}^{ext} - {}^{t}\mathbf{f}^{int} + \mathbf{M}\left(\frac{4}{\Delta t}\,{}^{t}\dot{\mathcal{U}} + {}^{t}\ddot{\mathcal{U}}\right) + \mathbf{D}\left(2\,{}^{t}\dot{\mathcal{U}}\right) \tag{5.60}$$

the equation to be solved for $\mathrm{d}\mathcal{U}$ can be written as

$$\mathbf{A}\mathrm{d}\mathcal{U} = \mathbf{b} \tag{5.61}$$

We note that in contrast to the above formulation for the implicit Euler scheme, the linear system is formulated in terms of displacements. As we will see in the upcoming section, this allows to easily incorporate movement constraints.

5.3.3. Projection based displacement constraints

We have already seen that Neumann boundary conditions are naturally included in the FE formulation through the external forces $\mathbf{f}^{ext}$. In contrast, displacement constraints have to be explicitly handled. Although it is rather difficult to prescribe displacement constraints at arbitrary points in $\mathcal{B}$ [BLM00], displacement constraints at the element nodes can be incorporated in a very computationally efficient way. In the following paragraph we present how to achieve this when the presented Newmark time integration scheme is used.
If the displacement $\overline{\mathcal{U}}_k$ of certain nodes $P_k, k \in \mathcal{S}$ in the set $\mathcal{S}$ is already known, the dimension of the linear system (5.61) is essentially reduced by the size of $\mathcal{S}$. However, in order to conserve matrix symmetry, the size of the linear system is usually not changed. Instead, the displacements are built into the system by a procedure that is called *displacement projection* (see Alg. 1). The core idea is to project the nodal displacements to the given values (i.e. set $\mathcal{U}_k = \overline{\mathcal{U}}_k \quad \forall k \in \mathcal{S}$) and then modify the linear system in such a way that for the result $\mathrm{d}\mathcal{U}_k = 0 \quad \forall k \in \mathcal{S}$.

5.4. Quadratic corotated tetrahedra

Having established the foundations of FE techniques, a computationally efficient soft tissue model based on corotated quadratic tetrahedra will be presented in this section. The formulation of the method as well as its extensive numerical validation for real-time deformable models and non-rigid registration is based on the respective proceedings publications [SRD+11] [SLH+13].

Algorithm 1 Newmark timestep with projection constraints

Project nodal displacements, i.e. set $\mathcal{U}_k = \overline{\mathcal{U}}_k \; \forall k \in \mathcal{S}$
Compute ${}^t\mathbf{f}^{int}$
Compute effective load $\mathbf{b}$ according to eq. 5.60
Project $\mathbf{b}$, i.e. set $\mathbf{b}_k = 0 \; \forall k \in \mathcal{S}$
Compute system matrix $\mathbf{A}$ according to eq. 5.59
Project $\mathbf{A}$, i.e. set k-th row and k-th column of $\mathbf{A}$ to 0 and $\mathbf{A}_k k = 1 \; \forall k \in \mathcal{S}$
Solve $\mathbf{A} d\mathcal{U} = \mathbf{b}$
Update displacements and velocities according to eq. 5.58

5.4.1. Corotated finite elements

As previously discussed, linear elastic models cannot be used if an object is subjected to large deformations, regardless of the material properties (linear deformation measures are not rotation invariant). However, if a fully non-linear formulation is used in a static setting or in conjunction with implicit time integration techniques, a non-linear system of equations has to be solved for each time step (see eq. 5.53). Corotated finite elements offer an attractive alternative to this computationally expensive approach and have become a popular choice for real-time deformable models in the realm of computer graphics. The core idea is to linearize the equation of motion by performing the polar decomposition (section 4.1.3)

$$\mathbf{F} = \mathbf{R}\mathbf{U} \tag{5.62}$$

of the deformation gradient $\mathbf{F}$ and using the stretch matrix $\mathbf{U}$ as the deformation measure. In this way a rotation-invariant formulation is achieved. Corotated FE are usually formulated in terms of the current nodal positions and the reference nodal positions, which are denoted by

$$\mathcal{X} = {}^t\mathcal{X} \qquad \text{and} \qquad \mathcal{X}_0 = {}^0\mathcal{X} \tag{5.63}$$

Technically speaking, all occurrences of the deformation gradient φ are substituted by the stretch matrix $\mathbf{U}$. In the following section we briefly show how the complete corotated FE approach emerges through this approach. For a detailed derivation we refer to the appendix A.6. The corotated Cauchy strain tensor can be formulated as

$$\epsilon^{CR} = \frac{1}{2}\left(\mathbf{R}^T \mathcal{X}_J \nabla N_J + (\mathbf{R}^T \mathcal{X}_J \nabla N_J)^T\right) - \mathbf{I} \tag{5.64}$$

The corotated stress σ^{CR} is then computed by inserting the corotated strain tensor into the material law eq. (4.99). The corotated nodal forces

$$\mathbf{f}^{int} = \int_{\Omega_0} R_{im} \sigma^{CR}_{mk} (\nabla N)_{kI} \mathrm{dV}_0 \tag{5.65}$$

can be derived accordingly and the corotated tangent stiffness matrix is

$$\mathbf{K}^{CR} = \sum_e \int_\tau \frac{\partial \hat{f}^{X,int}_{iI}}{\partial \mathcal{X}_{jJ}} \mathrm{dV}_0 = \sum_e \int_\tau \mathbf{R} \frac{\partial \hat{\mathbf{f}}^{int}_I}{\partial \mathcal{X}_J} \mathbf{R}^T \mathrm{dV}_0. \tag{5.66}$$

The approach can be described as rotating the deformation field into the initial configuration, calculating the nodal forces using the linear Cauchy strain tensor and finally rotating the forces back to the deformed configuration. By inserting the corotated nodal forces and the corotated stiffness matrix into eq. (5.53), we can finally express the implicit equilibrium:

$$\mathbf{M}\ddot{\mathcal{U}} + \mathbf{D}\mathrm{d}\dot{\mathcal{U}} + \mathbf{K}^{CR}\mathrm{d}\mathcal{U} = \mathbf{f}^{ext} - \mathbf{f}^{int} \tag{5.67}$$

At his point, an important difference to the full non-linear formulation has to be emphasized. When solving for the fully non-linear formulation, a sufficient number of Newton-Raphson steps have to be used in order for the simulation to remain stable. In contrast, the corotated form remains stable when only one Newton-Raphson step is performed each time step. Furthermore, the extraction of the rotational component changes the condition number of the element matrices only marginally which renders the simulation very stable. Although the method cannot model material non-linearities, it offers a very efficient way to achieve a geometrically non-linear formulation. However, in contrast to the linear FEM, the rotation matrices have to be computed and assembled into the stiffness matrix every time step.

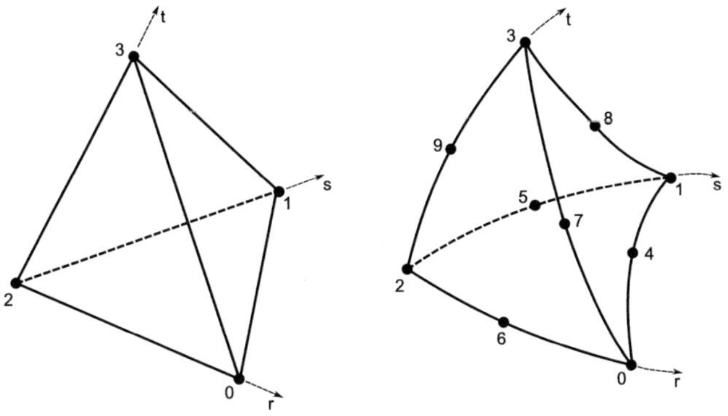

Figure 5.2.: Linear tetrahedron with 4 nodes (tet4) and quadratic tetrahedron with 10 nodes (tet10)

5.4.2. Quadratic tetrahedra

The isoparametric 4-node tetrahedron interpolates the position linearly between the nodes (Fig. 5.2). Consequently, the stress is constant over the element and the element shows significant volumetric locking for nearly incompressible materials [BLM00]. In contrast, the 10-node tetrahedron interpolates positions with 2nd order polynomials and doesn't suffer from severe volume locking. Thus, in the realm of mechanical engineering it is well known that quadratic tetrahedra perform much better than linear tetrahedral meshes in many scenarios [CK92]. This is especially true for the simulation of incompressible objects.
Typically, the shape functions are defined in a local coordinate system (r,s,t) and all element based operations such as calculating deformations, extracting rotations or numerical integration are performed in this local coordinate system. Polynomial functions (*shape functions*) are used to map the local coordinates to the global coordinate system. If the polynomial degree of the shape functions matches the order of the basis functions, the element is called isoparametric. In case of the isoparametric 10-node tetrahedron, the shape functions are quadratic, which allows curved boundaries and therefore better approximation of the geometry (Fig. 5.2).

As previously mentioned, the integrals that arise during the computation of the forces and the stiffness matrix are evaluated numerically. One cubature point per element is sufficient in order to integrate the stiffness matrix term eq. (5.66) if linear basis functions are used. In contrast, four sample points are necessary to integrate the 10-node tetrahedron. Consequently, four rotation matrices have to be extracted per element for accurate integration. Alternatively, it is possible to extract just one rotation matrix per element by only using the four corner vertices in order to compute the deformation gradient. In this case the element matrix can be pre-computed and the numerical integration can be omitted, which reduces the computational costs by 75%. This simplification will be referred to as the single rotation quadratic tetrahedron.

5.4.3. Numerical validation

Numerical simulation studies on a simple beam geometry are performed in order to compare the efficiency of the linear tetrahedral (tet4), the quadratic tetrahedral (tet10) as well as the single rotation quadratic tetrahedral (tet10SR) elements. In the first scenario, the beam deforms under gravity, while it is subjected to a twisting deformation pattern in the second scenario (Fig. 5.3). Incompressible material models (Poisson's ration $\nu = 0.49$) are used throughout the study. The linear and the quadratic corotated FEM were implemented using the Simulation Open Framework Architecture (SOFA) toolkit [FDD+12]. For all simulations in this study, the Newmark time integration scheme is used along with the Pardiso direct sparse solver from the Intel MKL 10.3.
In order to perform a quantitative analysis of the discretization error for each model, a reference solution on a high resolution quadratic mesh (100k elements) is computed for both problems. Test models of different resolutions are subsequently compared to this reference model. We choose the root mean squared (RMS) error at the nodes of the reference solution as the error measures. The RMS errors with respect to the degrees of freedom (DOF) are depicted in Fig. 5.4.
In case of the gravity induced deformation, tet4 elements need much more DOF (up to 40x) than tet10 elements in order to achieve the same accuracy. This result illustrates the locking behavior of linear tetrahedral elements. It should also be pointed out that the tet10SR formulation shows only negligible difference to the fully integrated tet10 element.

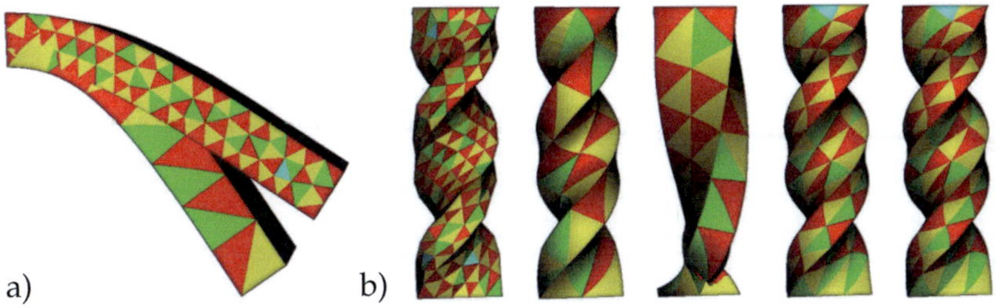

Figure 5.3.: Deformation under gravity (a) and twisting deformation pattern of a beam (b). A 1461 DOF tet4 mesh is compared to a 714 DOF tet10 mesh. The tet10SR element fails to capture the rotation at low resolution (b, middle), but achieves similar accuracy to the tet10 element at higher resolution (b, right).

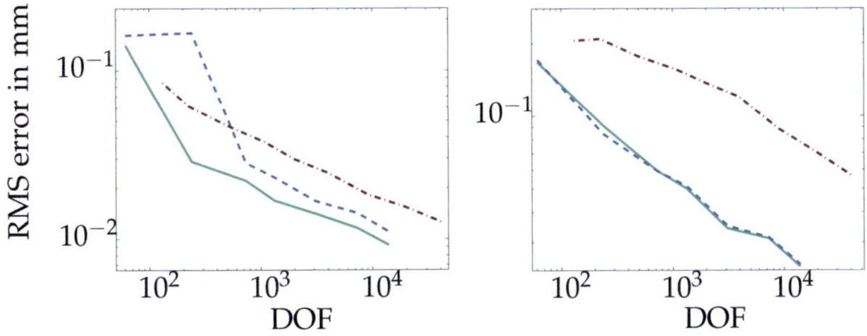

Figure 5.4.: RMS error over DOF for twisting deformation (left) and gravity induced deformation (right). The tet10 (green) and tet10SR (blue) elements show far superior accuracy for the same DOF than the tet4 (red) mesh.

Due to the displacement boundary conditions and the absence of volumetric forces, the difference in the twisting scenario is not as pronounced. However, the tet4 elements still need an order of magnitude more DOFs. It is apparent from Fig. 5.3 that the tet4 mesh with 1461 DOFs still shows visible edges, while the lower resolution tet10 mesh (714 DOFs) produces a smooth deformation. It can also be seen that the tet10SR element fails to capture the rotations at low resolution (Fig. 5.3), but achieves a

similar accuracy as the tet10 element for higher resolutions (right). It can be concluded that quadratic elements are superior to tet4 elements in both scenarios. Furthermore, the single rotation quadratic tetrahedral formulation (tet10SR) can be a computationally efficient alternative to the standard tet10 formulation for many applications.
We now compare the registration accuracy of the corotated formulation with the accuracy of a complex fully non-linear QLV model. For this purpose, we set up a similar simulation study as already presented in section 4.3.2. Here, we use a FE model with 8744 tet10 elements (14712 nodes) and use comparable boundary conditions as in the previous study (see Fig. 4.6). For the respiratory motion pattern scenario, the liver is deformed over a timespan of three seconds with a maximal displacement of 43.6 mm. The maximal displacement for the instrument indentation simulation is 11.07 mm. The QLV model by Raghunathan et al. [RES10] was again chosen as the reference model which was solved using the commercial FEM software ABAQUS.
It is apparent from table 5.1 that the maximal Euclidean distance (measured at the nodes of the meshes) between the corotated model and the QLV model is 0.47 mm for the respiratory deformation pattern. For the instrument indentation, the corotated model and the linear model achieve a similar accuracy (Table. 5.2).

Table 5.1.: Errors in comparison to a complex QLV model, respiratory deformation pattern

	Mean error [mm]	Max error [mm]	Standard deviation [mm]
Corotated model	0.13	0.47	0.08
Linear model	0.76	3.1	0.48

Table 5.2.: Errors in comparison to a complex QLV model, instrument indentation

	Mean error [mm]	Max error [mm]	Standard deviation [mm]
Corotated model	0.09	0.55	0.08
Linear model	0.03	0.65	0.04

Due to the fact that the linear model cannot adequately capture the large rotational components of the respiratory deformation pattern, it produces large errors in this case. In contrast, the solutions of the corotated model stay very close to the fully non-linear QLV model in both scenarios. Thus, we again demonstrate that the accurate solution of the displacement-zero traction boundary value problem necessarily requires a geometric non-linear formulation, while the material non-linearity is not that important.

It should be emphasized that this result holds, because the registration procedure can be described as a displacement-zero traction problem. Furthermore, the intraoperative navigation system does not have to capture the very rapid soft tissue deformations in order to provide a meaningful guidance. Both assumptions might not be fulfilled in the case of surgical simulation. In these scenarios one might be interested in calculating accurate feedback forces, which would require fully non-linear models.

5.5. Distributed computing for intraoperative real-time image guidance

Real-time intraoperative guidance is a computationally challenging problem. Different components such as image processing, registration and visualizations algorithms have to be integrated into a single system. In this context, the question arises how the components can be distributed over different workstations. Furthermore, it has to be investigated if distributed computation can in fact speed up computer assisted surgery (CAS) systems, or if the additional communication overhead actually reduces the performance of the system.

Here, we present a lightweight approach to distribute the workload over several workstations based on the OpenIGTLink protocol. In the following sections the basic approach is outlined and its application for biomechanically based soft tissue registration is discussed. For further details concerning the method as well as other applications please refer to the original publication [SKW+12].

5.5.1. OpenIGTLink based message passing

The OpenIGTLink protocol has been developed to share different data types such as image or positional data between intraoperative sensors and CAS workstations over a standard Ethernet connection [TFP+09]. The protocol has since emerged as an open source industry standard and has also been used to send commands to a robot control unit [TFD+10].
Several native data types such as images, transforms, positional and point data are already included in the standard OpenIGTLink protocol specification. The protocol has also been extended to support the transmission of XML messages [TFD+10]. It is thus possible to transmit all data types that can be encoded into XML. This approach is very flexible and well suited for small data sizes. However, it can be very slow if larger amounts of data such as FE meshes have to be transmitted in real-time. Therefore, we extended the OpenIGTLink protocol to natively support mesh and boundary condition data.
In order to control distributed CAS components, OpenIGTLink was extended to support XML-based remote method invocation. For this purpose a registry is used to allow an easy instantiation of remote objects. It assigns a unique identifier to each remote object upon creation. The connection manager can then relay each XML message to the appropriate receiver using this identifier. The method's arguments can be encoded directly into the XML message. Arguments that consist of large amounts of data can alternatively be sent as a follow-up message in a native data format in order to reduce the transmission overhead.

5.5.2. Timing measurements

The presented approach is used to run a finite element based soft tissue registration on a remote workstation. During a set-up process, the initial FE mesh is transferred from the primary CAS workstation to the simulation server. For every time step, the boundary conditions are subsequently transferred to the remote server while the deformed mesh is sent back to the CAS server after each simulation step is completed. We measure both the total execution time on the CAS workstation and the total simulation time on the simulation server. The pure transmission is thus given by the difference of these measurements.

Table 5.3.: Transmission times for different mesh sizes using XML-based message passing.

DOF	Size [byte]	Transmission time [ms]
72	11,350	2.9
291	45,127	7.1
1113	156,613	26.3
5430	728,568	100.4
13863	1,809,506	218.1
26970	3,527,806	415.4
57384	7,494,936	814.7
136254	17,746,520	2061.5

Table 5.4.: Transmission times for different mesh sizes using native data types.

DOF	Size [byte]	Transmission time [ms]
72	2,048	1.0
291	8,092	1.3
1113	28,164	2.0
5430	129,432	6.0
13863	320,684	13.7
26970	618,408	26.1
57384	1,300,592	50.2
136254	3,062,696	119.2

As it should be expected, the transmission time is linear in terms of the number of degrees of freedom (DOFs) for both the XML-based and the native data types (Table 5.3 and 5.4). The transmission time of the XML-encoded data is rather high as the moderately sized meshes with 5430 DOF cannot be transmitted in real-time (100.4 ms transmission time). In contrast, the native encoding reduces the transmission time by more than an order of magnitude. The delay for the 5430 DOF mesh is thus reduced to 6ms. This transmission time is not only compatible with real-time constraints, but also much lower than the computation time on a single core CPU. The large difference between the two encoding modes can be attributed to the significantly larger size of the XML-encoded data.

Also, the parsing of the XML message is significantly slower than the unpacking of the native encoding.
If highly optimized FE algorithms are run on GPU-accelerated workstation (please refer to the following chapter for details), the transmission time can become significant in comparison to the total execution time. However, it has to be pointed out that the whole deformed mesh was sent back to the CAS workstation in the presented experiments. In a typical application, the transmitted data could be optimized by only transferring necessary data such as tumor or vessel locations.

5.5.3. Discussion

It has been demonstrated that corotated elasticity models are well suited for real-time soft tissue registration. In addition, it has become apparent that quadratic corotated tetrahedra severely outperform linear tetrahedra in terms of accuracy per degrees of freedom. Finally, it was shown how a FE based registration algorithm for a CAS applications can be moved to a dedicated workstation.
However, even if the FE simulation does not have to share computing resources with other CAS components, a straight forward CPU implementation only allows simulating a few hundred tet10 elements in real-time. For many registration applications larger model sizes are required in order to obtain a sufficient accuracy.
In the next chapter we will see how an efficient GPU-based finite element solver can be used to significantly increase the complexity of the real-time model. For this purpose, a highly parallel multigrid solving scheme will be presented. Furthermore it will be shown how complex geometries can be accurately embedded into low-resolution quadratic tetrahedral meshes.

Science is what we understand well enough to explain to a computer. Art is everything else we do.

— Donald E. Knuth

6. Fast GPU-based finite element solver

In this chapter, we present a set of novel methods to efficiently simulate corotated quadratic FE models in real-time. First, we address the problem how high resolution surface meshes can be mapped to quadratic isoparametric elements. In this scenario, the difficulty arises from the fact that the mapping from the reference element to each quadratic element is not bijective and not analytically invertible. Furthermore, there are far less elements in a higher order FE mesh than in a linear mesh if compared in terms of DOF. Therefore, it becomes more important to accurately extrapolate deformations to surface points outside the FE mesh. In this chapter, we present a novel mapping scheme to overcome this problem.

Massively parallel hardware (so called general purpose graphics processing units - GPGPU) have become a popular choice in recent years for speeding up time-critical algorithms in the realm of image processing and simulation. Although this hardware type offers a significantly higher performance in terms of floating point operations per second than traditional CPU architectures, the algorithms have to be carefully designed in order to fully exploit these resources. In particular, the algorithm has to be heavily parallelizable. In the following, an efficient GPU based solver for quadratic corotated tetrahedra is presented. For this purpose, we first introduce a matrix-free scheme in order to facilitate the implementation of a GPU based conjugate gradient (CG) solver. Then, we show how the performance of this solver can be greatly enhanced by using a parallel preconditioner based on the factorized sparse approximate inverse (FSAI). Finally, we present a novel GPU-based multigrid scheme to efficiently solve elasticity models on higher order, unstructured, non-conforming grids.

6.1. Accurate surface embedding for higher order finite elements

In this section a novel approach to accurately map highly detailed surface meshes to a higher order FE computational mesh is presented. The novel mapping scheme relies on a representation of each surface vertex in terms of a point on the computational mesh and its distance to the FE mesh in normal direction. Through this representation, the surface deformations remain smooth and local shape features are preserved even if very low-resolution FE meshes are used for computation. An efficient algorithm based on non-linear optimization is proposed to construct the mapping. We show that the algorithm performs robustly and that its numerical complexity is linear in the number of surface nodes and constant in the number nodes in the computational mesh.
The following description and evaluation of the novel mapping scheme is based on the corresponding proceedings publication [SLH+13].

6.1.1. Closest point search in higher order meshes

In order to facilitate the computation of the mapping later on, we first detail an efficient scheme to compute the closest point $\mathbf{p}(r,s,t)$ in the FE mesh $\mathcal{M}$ for each vertex v of the triangular surface mesh $\mathcal{S}$. We will first show how to find $\mathbf{p}(r,s,t)$ for a single given vertex v. Based on this results, a recursive mapping scheme will be introduced that can be used to compute $\mathbf{p}(r,s,t)$ for all v in $\mathcal{S}$.
The distance $d(r,s,t)$ from a point $\mathbf{p}(r,s,t)$ in the element τ to an arbitrary surface vertex v is given by

$$d(r,s,t) = \|v - \mathbf{x}_I N_I(r,s,t)\| . \tag{6.1}$$

As ν can be outside of τ, we have to constrict (r,s,t) such that $\mathbf{p}(r,s,t)$ is indeed in τ. We can thus formulate the closest point search in terms of the constrained optimization problem

$$\begin{aligned} &\min d(\mathbf{p}(r,s,t)) \quad \text{s.t.} \\ &r > 0, s > 0, t > 0 \quad \text{and} \quad r+s+t \leq 1. \end{aligned} \tag{6.2}$$

As previously mentioned, the solution to this problem can be analytically determined if linear shape functions are used. For higher order shape functions, non-linear programming techniques have to be employed. We solve the constrained optimization problem (eq. X6.2) using an extended Levenberg-Marquardt algorithm [NW99] [KYF05]. The Jacobian is calculated using finite differences. It is important to point out that simple Newton-Raphson iterations are not guaranteed to converge even in the unconstrained case when ν is inside τ.
The solution to problem (6.2) can be described as the local optimum for $\mathbf{p}(r,s,t) \in \tau$. The next step is to find the element $\tau_{\min}$ where $\mathbf{p}(r,s,t)$ reaches its global minimum distance $d_{\min}$ in $\mathcal{M}$. This can be efficiently accomplished with a recursive algorithm (see algorithm 2).
We first select an element τ to start the iteration. Subsequently the closest point $\mathbf{p} \in \tau$ to ν is computed. This procedure is recursively called on the neighboring tetrahedra, if $\mathbf{p}$ is on a face of τ. The recursion is aborted if $d = 0$ (i.e. $\mathbf{p}$ is inside the current tetrahedron) or if the neighbor tetrahedron that shares the face has already been visited (i.e. is in set $\mathcal{T}$). During each recursion step, the minimum distance $d_{\min}$ in $\tau_{\min}$ is updated if a closer point $\hat{\mathbf{p}}$ is found.
The algorithm efficiently computes the local minimum distance $d_{\min}$ for a given initial guess τ. This local minimum coincides with the global minimum if the initial guess τ is close enough to the real solution.

6.1.2. Recursive mapping scheme

We now seek to not only map the whole surface mesh $\mathcal{S}$ to the computation grid, but also to reliable find the global minimum $d_{\min}$ for all $\tau_i \in \mathcal{M}$. For this purpose we introduce an outer recursion to the presented algorithm 2. An initial mapping correspondence is established by finding the closest surface vertex ν_0 in $\mathcal{S}$ for an arbitrary point $\mathbf{p}_0$ in τ_0. It is important to point out that this inverse mapping problem is much

Algorithm 2 Recursively find $\mathbf{p}(r,s,t) \in \mathcal{M}$

```
procedure ClosestPoint(ν, τ, d_min, τ_min, 𝒯)
    Solve (6.2) to find closest point p with distance d
    to ν in τ
    if d < d_min then
        d_min = d, τ_min = τ
    if p is on face of τ then
        if p is on surface of ℳ then
            if p is on surface edge then
                Find neighbour tetrahedron τ_1 that contains
                surface triangle which shares edge
        else
            Find tetrahedron τ_1 that shares face
        if τ_1 exists and τ_1 ∉ 𝒯 then
            Add τ_1 to 𝒯
            (p̂, d̂, τ̂) = ClosestPoint(ν, τ_1, d_min, τ_min, 𝒯)
            if d̂ < d_min then
                d = d̂, τ = τ̂, p = p̂
                d_min = d, τ_min = τ
    return p, d, τ
```

easier to solve as the resolution of $\mathcal{S}$ is much higher than the resolution of $\mathcal{M}$.

In order to start the outer recursion, we arbitrarily select an initial triangle $\mathbb{T}_0$ that contains ν_0. We than start a recursive scheme which maps all points in a given triangle $\mathbb{T}$ and uses the current mapping results $(\mathbf{p}, \tau)$ as the initial guess for mapping the neighbor triangles of $\mathbb{T}$ (see algorithm 3).

The initial guess for each triangle depends on the mapping order of the triangles. Thus, there might be mapping orders that don't generate initial guesses which guarantee a global optimum for $d_{\min}$. That's why the mapping order is controlled by introducing the distance threshold d_t. The triangle $\mathbb{T}$ is only mapped (and the recursion only continues) if the distance for each surface vertex in $\mathbb{T}$ is below d_t. In order to make sure

Algorithm 3 Recursively map triangles in $\mathcal{S}$

```
procedure MapTriangle(𝕋, τ, d_t, 𝒫)
    triangleMapped = true
    for all Surface vertices ν in 𝕋 do
        if ν ∉ 𝒫 then
            Initialize empty 𝒯, d_min = inf
            (p, d, τ̂) = ClosestPoint(ν, τ, d_min, τ_min, 𝒯)
            if d < d_t then
                τ = τ̂
                Map vertex ν to point p in τ
                Add ν to 𝒫
            else
                triangleMapped = false
    if triangleMapped then
        for all Neigbour triangles 𝕋_n do
            MapTriangle(𝕋_i, τ, d_t, 𝒫)
    return
```

that all triangles are mapped, this distance threshold is incrementally raised until all triangles are mapped.
For implementation purposes, the recursive scheme has to be unrolled into a loop in order to ensure an efficient and stable computation for large meshes.

6.1.3. Accurate surface embedding

We now define a scheme that maps the surface mesh $\mathcal{S}$ onto the computational mesh $\mathcal{M}$ such that the deformed surface $\mathcal{S}'$ can be extrapolated from the deformed FE mesh $\mathcal{M}'$ in a fast and correct way. For this purpose we represent each surface model vertex ν in terms of a point $\mathbf{p}$ on the FE grid and its distance d in normal direction (see Fig. 6.1). The deformed vertex position

$$\nu' = \mathbf{p}' + d\mathbf{n}' \tag{6.3}$$

can subsequently be constructed using the position of $\mathbf{p}$ in the deformed configuration ($\mathbf{p}'$) as well as the deformed normal $\mathbf{n}'$. It will become

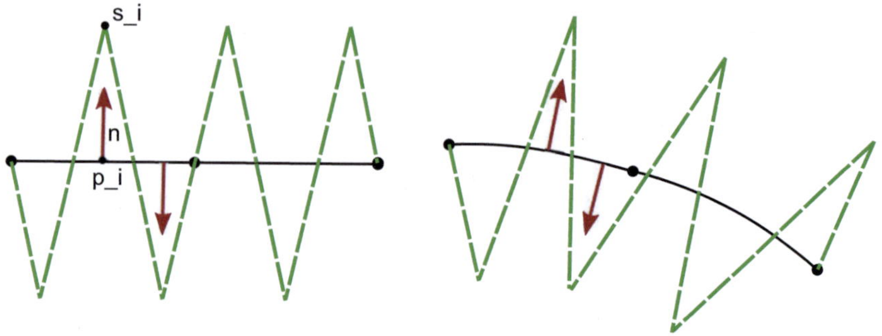

Figure 6.1.: Sawtooth surface attached to 1D quadratic edge. The deformation of the edge can be extrapolated to the surface while preserving local shape features.

apparent from the numerical examples that the proposed mapping preserves the smoothness of the deformation (and thus local shape features) even for surface regions that lie outside of the computational mesh.

6.1.4. Smooth normal field

At any surface point $\mathbf{p}$ on the mesh given in local coordinates r,s with respect to the quadratic surface triangle, the spatial derivatives

$$\frac{\partial \mathbf{x}(\mathbf{p})}{\partial r} = \mathbf{x}_I \frac{\partial N_I(r,s)}{\partial r} \quad , \quad \frac{\partial \mathbf{x}(\mathbf{p})}{\partial s} = \mathbf{x}_I \frac{\partial N_I(r,s)}{\partial s} \tag{6.4}$$

can be calculated using the position of the nodes and the shape function derivatives at r,s of the 6 node quadratic triangle. The normal $\mathbf{n}$ at $\mathbf{p}$ is then given by

$$\mathbf{n} = \left(\frac{\partial \mathbf{x}(\mathbf{p})}{\partial r} \times \frac{\partial \mathbf{x}(\mathbf{p})}{\partial s} \right) / \left\| \frac{\partial \mathbf{x}(\mathbf{p})}{\partial r} \times \frac{\partial \mathbf{x}(\mathbf{p})}{\partial s} \right\| . \tag{6.5}$$

A smooth normal field is a necessary condition for the smoothness of the proposed mapping scheme. As the FE mesh is only C^0-continuous, the partial derivatives (and thus the normals) are discontinuous at element boundaries. Therefore, we average the normal at each node using the angle weighted average scheme. This results in an averaged normal $\overline{\mathbf{n}}_I$ for each surface vertex of the FE mesh and the normal

$$\mathbf{n} = (\overline{\mathbf{n}}_I N_I(r,s)) / \|\overline{\mathbf{n}}_I N_I(r,s)\| \tag{6.6}$$

can be interpolated using the standard shape functions of the quadratic triangle. The smooth normal field that is created in this way can be efficiently computed. Furthermore, it is not necessary to re-compute the deformed vertex normals $\overline{\mathbf{n}}'_I$ every time step as shown in eq. (6.5). Instead, nodal rotation matrices can be defined at each node of the FE mesh which can be used to rotate the normal into the deformed configuration.

6.1.5. Normal correction

The aforementioned representation of each surface vertex v in terms of $(\mathbf{p}, d)$ can be obtained by solving a global optimization problem. The solution to this problem is not necessarily unique for complex, non-convex meshes. In order to construct the representation we first find the closest point $\mathbf{p} \in \mathcal{M}$ to v. Due to the normal smoothing, the normal $\mathbf{n}$ at $\mathbf{p}$ does not necessarily point in the direction of v. Thus, we perform an additional correction step to make sure that the normal $\mathbf{n}$ at $\mathbf{p}$ does indeed point in the direction of v. For this purpose we define the difference vector

$$\delta(r,s,t) = v_i - (\mathbf{x}_I N_I(r,s,t) + d \cdot \overline{\mathbf{n}}_I N_I(r,s,t)), \tag{6.7}$$

where d denotes the distance as defined in eq. (6.1). The correction step can then be formulated in terms of the minimization problem

$$\begin{aligned} &\min \delta(r,s,t)\,\text{s.t.} \\ &r > 0, s > 0, t > 0\,\text{and}\, r + s + t \leq 1. \end{aligned} \tag{6.8}$$

The optimization problem is solved in the same way as problem (6.2): A recursive scheme along the lines of algorithm 2 is employed on top of a constrained Levenberg-Marquardt optimizer that uses finite differences to approximate the Jacobian.

6.2. Matrix free conjugate gradient solver

The necessary steps for solving the fully discretized scheme of the dynamic corotational formulation have already been outlined in section 5.3.3. From this scheme, three computationally significant steps can be extracted: The computation of the nodal forces, the assembly of the stiffness matrix and the linear system solve.
The nodal force computation consists of two stages. First, the elemental rotations are extracted and the elemental stiffness matrices are obtained through numerical integration. Afterwards, the elemental contributions are added to the nodal force vector. The whole process is inherently parallel and can be easily implemented on the GPU. In accordance with previous work (e.g. Allard et al. [ACF11]) we use one kernel launch to perform the elemental computations such as the polar decomposition of the deformation gradient and an additional kernel launch for the per-vertex gather operation.
Implementing the matrix assembly and system solve step on the GPU is much more difficult. Most linear solvers (in particular the direct ones) do not parallelize well. For symmetric and positive definite systems an exception exists in the form of the conjugate gradient (CG) approach. This iterative method describes the linear system solve as a minimization problem for convex quadratic functions. The core ideas is to use so called conjugate directions instead of the local gradient for an efficient gradient descent minimization scheme [NW99].
A basic sketch of the CG scheme (see Alg. 4) reveals that only simple computational tasks such as vector addition, vector-vector multiplication and a (sparse) matrix-vector product are necessary for the system solve. In the context of an efficient GPU implementation, the most challenging part is the sparse matrix-vector product (SpMV) between the system matrix (see eq. 5.61) and the current search direction p_k in each CG step. In order to avoid a time-consuming matrix assembly, we don't build the system matrix every time step, but instead use a similar approach as Allard et al. [ACF11]: We first compute the per-element contributions for each nodal force and then accumulate these results for each node. In contrast to Allard et al. (and in contrast to the procedure for computing the nodal forces), we don't use a separate kernel launch for the per-vertex operations. Instead, we use a multi-coloring technique such that primarily those elements who do not share a common node are processed

Algorithm 4 Conjugate gradient algorithm for solving $\mathbf{Ax} = \mathbf{b}$

set $\mathbf{x}_0 = 0, \mathbf{r}_0 = \mathbf{A}\mathbf{x}_0 - \mathbf{b}, \mathbf{p}_0 = -\mathbf{r}_0, k = 0$
for $k = 0 <$ maxIter **do**
  if $\|\mathbf{r}_k\| / \|\mathbf{b}\| < \epsilon$ **then**
    break
  $\alpha_k = \dfrac{\mathbf{r}_k^T \mathbf{r}_k}{\mathbf{Z}_k^T \mathbf{A} \mathbf{Z}_k}$
  $\mathbf{x}_{k+1} = \mathbf{x}_k + \alpha \mathbf{p}_k$
  $\mathbf{r}_{k+1} = \mathbf{x}_k + \alpha \mathbf{A} \mathbf{p}_k$
  $\beta_{k+1} = \dfrac{\mathbf{r}_{k+1}^T \mathbf{r}_{k+1}}{\mathbf{r}_k^T \mathbf{r}_k}$
  $\mathbf{Z}_{k+1} = -\mathbf{r}_{k+1} + \beta_{k+1} \mathbf{Z}_k$
  k=k+1

in parallel. With our layout it is still possible (although very rare) that the nodal force contributions of two elements of different color are updated simultaneously. We thus use an atomic operation in order to add these contributions to the nodal forces. As the atomic add causes virtually no overhead when no write conflicts occur, it is very efficient when used in combination with coloring techniques.
The elemental contributions are computed by multiplying dense elemental matrices with corresponding nodal vectors. The performance of this kernel is limited by the memory bandwidth. In order to reduce the data transfer to global memory and to reduce the amount of shared memory used by each thread, we exploit the symmetry of the elemental matrices and use compressed matrices for data transfer. The matrix vector product is then performed using a constant lookup table for index mapping between the compressed and the uncompressed matrix.

6.3. FSAI preconditioned conjugate gradients

For inhomogeneous and stiff materials, the discrete elasticity problem becomes increasingly ill-conditioned, i.e. the condition number

$$\kappa(\mathbf{A}) = \|\mathbf{A}\| \cdot \left\|\mathbf{A}^{-1}\right\| \tag{6.9}$$

becomes large. In this case, pure CG methods converge very poorly. A proven solution to this problem is to apply a preconditioner $\mathbf{Z}$[1] to the linear system. It is immediatly clear from

$$\mathbf{Z}^{-1}\mathbf{A}\mathbf{dx} = \mathbf{Z}^{-1}\mathbf{b} \tag{6.10}$$

that if $\mathbf{Z}^{-1}$ is close to $\mathbf{A}$, then $\mathbf{Z}^{-1}\mathbf{A}$ is near the identity matrix and the condition number κ is low. If a preconditioner is used in a CG scheme, it has to be applied in each iteration, i.e. the equation

$$\mathbf{Zr} = \mathbf{z} \tag{6.11}$$

has to be solved for the temporary vector $\mathbf{r}$ and the right hand side $\mathbf{z}$. That is why a key requirement for a good preconditioner is that its application according to eq. (6.11) is fast and efficient. The Jacobi preconditioner therefore simply scales $\mathbf{A}$ with its inverse diagonal which means it uses the preconditioner $\mathbf{Z} = \text{diag}(\mathbf{A})$.
A family of powerful preconditioners arises from the decomposition of $\mathbf{A}$ into triangular matrices. Every arbitrary square matrix can be written as the product of a lower and upper triangular matrix (LU decomposition). For symmetric, positive definite matrices the incomplete Cholesky (IC) decomposition

$$\mathbf{A} \approx \mathbf{L}_A\mathbf{L}_A^T = \mathbf{Z} \tag{6.12}$$

can drastically reduce the number of CG iterations for elastic problems [CAD+10]. The application of the IC preconditioner requires two triangular solves of the sparse triangular matrices $\mathbf{L}_A, \mathbf{L}_A^T$. While this can be very efficient on the CPU, the triangular solve is inherently recursive, which makes a GPU implementation difficult.
The factorized sparse approximate inverse (FSAI) preconditioner is based on a different idea [KY93]. This method seeks to directly approximate the inverse of $\mathbf{A}$. In order to achieve this goal, $\mathbf{A}^{-1}$ is decomposed according to

$$\mathbf{A}^{-1} \approx \mathbf{G}_L^T\mathbf{G}_L = \mathbf{Z}^{-1}. \tag{6.13}$$

In this context, the matrix $\mathbf{G}_L$ is an approximation the inverse of the lower Cholesky factor $\mathbf{L}_A$ in terms of the Frobenius norm $\|\mathbf{I} - \mathbf{G}_L\mathbf{L}_A\|_F$.

[1] often denoted with **P** in the literature, we use **Z** to avoid confusion with the first Piola-Kirchhoff stress tensor

The approximation is constructed by minimizing the aforementioned Frobenius norm for a given sparsity pattern of $\mathbf{G}_L$. The commonly used FSAI(q) method uses the sparsity pattern of $|\mathbf{A}|^q$.
The application of the FSAI preconditioner only needs two SpMV operations which are very fast on the GPU. It is clear that the more fill-ins are allowed in a higher order FSAI(q) scheme, the better is the approximation to $\mathbf{A}^{-1}$. However, at the same time the SpMV becomes increasingly time-consuming to compute.
The biggest drawback of the FSAI preconditioner is its high set-up time. In the next section we describe how to overcome this problem.

6.3.1. Preconditioner warping

In the context of interactive simulations it is not feasible to compute the preconditioner every timestep, especially if complex schemes such as IC or FSAI are used. A better strategy is to compute the preconditioner just once and then appropriately adapt it every time step. For elasticity problems based on the corotated formulation, this can be efficiently achieved by local rotation warping of the preconditioner [CAD+10]. The idea is based on the fact that the change in the system matrix $\mathbf{A}$ is dominated by the rotation warping of the elemental stiffness matrices (eq. 5.66).
In order to apply these rotations to $\mathbf{Z}^{-1}$, we extract a local rotation $\mathbf{R}_n$ per node. We can subsequently define the global block diagonal rotation matrix $\mathbf{R}$ to formulate

$$\mathbf{R}\mathbf{Z}^{-1}\mathbf{R}^T\mathbf{A}\mathbf{dx} = \mathbf{R}\mathbf{Z}^{-1}\mathbf{R}^T\mathbf{b}. \tag{6.14}$$

It is important to note that we do not have to explicitly compute $\mathbf{R}\mathbf{Z}^{-1}\mathbf{R}^T$ for each timestep, instead we serially apply the three operators. In this case it is not even necessary to build the global matrix $\mathbf{R}$, but each node can instead be rotated using the 3×3 matrix $\mathbf{R}_n$.
In the corotated FE model, the rotations are extracted on a per element basis. In order to compute the nodal rotations, we average the elemental rotations for each element around the node. This is done by first averaging the deformation gradient at the node before performing the rotation extraction according to Higham et al. [HS88]. We have found this procedure to be more efficient than directly averaging the rotations

using quaternions. In the case of quadratic tetrahedra, we use only the 4 corner vertices to compute the deformation gradient as explained in section 5.4.2.
Thanks to the warping scheme, the FSAI preconditioner can be computed in a pre-processing step from the linear stiffness matrix. It is even possible to store the preconditioner to disk and just load it at the beginning of each simulation.
The GPU implementation of the rotation warping and the subsequent application of the FSAI preconditioner is straight forward as the process is inherently parallel with a high data locality. As described above the rotation warping is performed by simply multiplying each node with a 3×3 rotation matrix. The application of the FSAI preconditioner requires two SpMV products. As the FSAI matrices do not change during the simulation, we just store them in GPU memory and apply them using a suitable CUDA library.

6.4. GPU-based multigrid solver for unstructured, non-conforming meshes

The computational effort for the preconditioned conjugate gradient approach does scale superlinearly in terms of the number of mesh nodes (i.e. the DOF): Not only does the computational time for each PCG iteration increase, but the number of PCG steps increases as well for a fixed residual threshold. Thus, the method becomes inefficient for high resolution models. In contrast, multigrid methods can keep the computational effort proportional to the number of mesh nodes. The core idea is to efficiently remove low frequency errors by solving the linear system on a hierarchy of grids with different resolutions.
In this section, we present a novel multigrid scheme for efficiently solving elasticity problems using higher order FE on unstructured, non-conforming grids. We furthermore outline a set of methods that allows to efficiently implement the scheme on massively parallel architectures. In the following, we first give a brief general introduction to geometric multigrid schemes for solving linear systems that arise from elliptic PDEs. In this context we especially highlight the necessary components of the approach. Based on this discussion, we present a suitable pro-

longation/restriction scheme and a highly parallel smoothing scheme for simulations on unstructured grids. Finally, we detail a multigrid-preconditioned CG solver for the real-time simulation of deformable models.

6.4.1. Basic multigrid scheme

At the core of a multigrid solver lies a hierarchy of problem discretizations of different resolutions. This hierarchy consists of $l_{\max}$ levels with the associated system matrices $\mathbf{A}_l$. The solution scheme starts with an initial guess $\mathbf{x}_0$ on level $l = 0$. In practice $\mathbf{x}_0$ is often chosen to be a vector of zeros or a value from a previous time step. The high frequency errors in this solution are subsequently attenuated by applying the smoothing operator $\mathcal{S}$. Typically, a variant of a fixed point iteration is used for this purpose (see section 6.4.3 for details). In order to eliminate the low frequency errors, the remaining residual is consequently transferred to the next level $l + 1$ with lower resolution. To do so, the residual $\mathbf{r}_l$ is first computed on the level l and then transferred to the lower resolution mesh using the restriction operator $\mathcal{R}$ (refer to section 6.4.2 for more information). If the maximal mesh level $l_{\max}$ is reached, the remaining error $\mathbf{e}_{l+1}$ is determined by solving $\mathbf{A}_{l+1}\mathbf{e}_{l+1} = \mathbf{r}_{l+1}$ on the coarser mesh. This can be either done with a direct solver or using an iterative method such as the previously presented preconditioned gradient approach. If $l + 1 < l_{\max}$, then the residual equation is recursively solved on the remaining levels of subsequently coarser meshes. In both cases, the error correction $\mathbf{e}_{l+1}$ is then transferred to the finer mesh at level l by means of the prolongation operator $\mathcal{P}$. After adding the correction term $\mathbf{e}_l$ to the solution, a final smoothing step removes high-frequency errors that are introduced by the prolongation process.
In practice, several variants of the described multigrid scheme are used. First of all, the number of levels $l_{\max}$ can vary depending on the application. Furthermore, the described V-cycle is usually repeated several times until a given residual threshold is met. Finally, in many applications it is more efficient to spend more solving time on the coarse grids, thus leading to so called W-cycles. For a more detailed discussion on the basics of geometric multigrid methods we refer to appropriate textbooks [Bra07].

Algorithm 5 V-cycle multigrid scheme for solving $\mathbf{Ax} = \mathbf{b}$

procedure MULTIGRIDSOLVE($\mathbf{x}_0, \mathbf{b}, l$)
  $\mathbf{x} \leftarrow \mathcal{S}(\mathbf{x}_0, \mathbf{A}_l, \mathbf{b})$
  $\mathbf{r}_l = \mathbf{A}_l \mathbf{x} - \mathbf{b}$
  $\mathbf{r}_{l+1} \leftarrow \mathcal{R}(\mathbf{r}_l)$
  if $l + 1 < l_{\max}$ **then**
    InnerSolve $\mathbf{A}_{l+1} \mathbf{e}_{l+1} = \mathbf{r}_{l+1}$
  else
    MultigridSolve($\mathbf{e}_{l+1}, \mathbf{b}_{l+1}, l + 1$)
  $\mathbf{e}_l \leftarrow \mathcal{P}(\mathbf{e}_{l+1})$
  $\mathbf{x} = \mathbf{x} + \mathbf{e}_l$
  $\mathbf{x} \leftarrow \mathcal{S}(\mathbf{x}, \mathbf{A}_l, \mathbf{b})$
  return $\mathbf{x}$

6.4.2. Multigrid hierarchy for non-conforming, higher order meshes

An accurate transfer of quantities between the meshes in the grid hierarchy is key in order to achieve an efficient multigrid scheme. For elasticity problems, the prolongation operator interpolates displacements between the meshes. The restriction operator transfers forces from a finer to a coarser grid. In many applications for geometric multigrid methods (especially in the realm of computational fluid mechanics), the finer mesh levels are constructed from an initial coarse mesh. In this way, all mesh levels cover the same region Ω_0 (conforming mesh hierarchy). A construction of suitable prolongation and restriction operators is thus straight forward. Typically, these operators are linear and therefore have a matrix representation. In this context, the restriction operator is often chosen to be the transpose of the prolongation scheme.
In order to accurately solve elasticity problems on unstructured grids, it is important to approximate the geometry as closely as possible. It is thus not desirable to construct the grid hierarchy from a coarse initial mesh. Instead, each mesh in the hierarchy should approximate the geometry as best as possible. Consequently, the meshes do not entirely overlap (non-conforming hierarchy) and thus displacements have to be

extrapolated. When using linear tetrahedral grids, this can be achieved using barycentric coordinates [GW08].
As outlined in section 6.1 the interpolation and extrapolation of displacement and force fields that are defined on higher order isoparametric grids is more challenging. In our multigrid scheme, we use the previously presented mapping scheme based on the surface normal in order to interpolate the displacement between meshes (prolongation). In order to restrict the residual force vector to a coarser mesh, we do not make use of the surface normal. Rather, we map each nodal force to the corresponding element τ in the coarse mesh that contains the closest point $\mathbf{p}(r,s,t)$ to the node. This force is then distributed among the nodes of τ according to the basis function values at $\mathbf{p}(r,s,t)$.

6.4.3. GPU-based smoothing

The smoothing operators that are commonly used in geometric multigrid solvers can be expressed as fixed point iteration schemes. The idea of this class of iterative methods is to use the non-singular matrix $\mathbf{B}$ in order to express the linear system $\mathbf{Ax} = \mathbf{b}$ through

$$\mathbf{Bx} + (\mathbf{A} - \mathbf{B})\mathbf{x} = \mathbf{b}. \tag{6.15}$$

The definition of the iteration

$$\mathbf{Bx}^{k+1} + (\mathbf{A} - \mathbf{B})\mathbf{x}^{k} = \mathbf{b} \tag{6.16}$$

yields the update equation

$$\mathbf{x}^{k+1} = \mathbf{x}^{k} - \mathbf{B}^{-1}(\mathbf{Ax}^{k} - \mathbf{b}). \tag{6.17}$$

By decomposing $\mathbf{A} = \mathbf{A}_D + \mathbf{A}_L + \mathbf{A}_U$ into the diagonal matrix $\mathbf{A}_D$ as well as the lower triangular matrix $\mathbf{A}_L$ and the upper triangular matrix $\mathbf{A}_U$, we can define two important smoothing schemes: Choosing $\mathbf{B} = \mathbf{A}_D$ yields the Jacobi method, while the Gauss-Seidel iteration scheme arises if $\mathbf{B} = \mathbf{A}_D + \mathbf{A}_L$. In a similar fashion as preconditioning techniques (see section 6.3), smoothing operators tend to work well, if $\mathbf{B}^{-1}$ is a good approximation of $\mathbf{A}^{-1}$. Thus, another class of commonly used smoothers are given by triangular decompositions of $\mathbf{A}$ such as $\mathbf{B} = \mathbf{LU}$ (incomplete LU factorization) or $\mathbf{B} = \mathbf{LL}^T$(incomplete Cholesky factorization).

It is apparent that the most efficient smoothers (e.g. Gauss-Seidel, ILU) rely on iteration schemes that are inherently recursive and thus not suitable for GPU implementation. For structured grids it is possible to divide the mesh into sets of non-neighboring elements (*mesh coloring*) in order to parallelize the Gauss-Seidel method. However, this approach is very inefficient on unstructured grids.
In order to facilitate a more efficient smoothing scheme, we use the previously presented FSAI technique ($\mathbf{B}^{-1} = \mathbf{G}_L^T \mathbf{G}_L$). We again choose to precompute this decomposition and use the rotation warping technique to update the smoothing matrix for each time step. This results in a highly parallel algorithm that can be efficiently implemented on the GPU. In order to compute the SpMV product in the update equation (6.17), we again use the presented matrix-free scheme in order to avoid an assembly of the global system matrix.

6.4.4. Multigrid-preconditioned CG for real-time elasticity

We found that in many low-resolution elasticity problems, the prolongation leads to larger high-frequency errors near Dirichlet boundaries. Consequently, many smoothing steps are necessary, if the multigrid scheme is directly used for solving the linear system. An attractive alternative is to use the multigrid scheme as a preconditioner in a PCG algorithm. In this case, the accuracy of the multigrid iterations can be intentionally reduced. Thus it is enough to perform one V-cycle and 1 or 2 smoothing iterations within each preconditioning step. In order to achieve an efficient GPU implementation, we use the previously presented FSAI-preconditioned CG solver to perform the inner solve. Here, a residual threshold as high as 0.1 can be used without significantly degrading the performance of the solver.

6.5. Performance evaluations

6.5.1. Accurate surface embedding

The novel mapping scheme was integrated into the SOFA framework [FDD$^+$12]. The constrained Levenberg-Marquardt implementation from the Levmar library was used to solve the minimization problem (eq. 6.2)

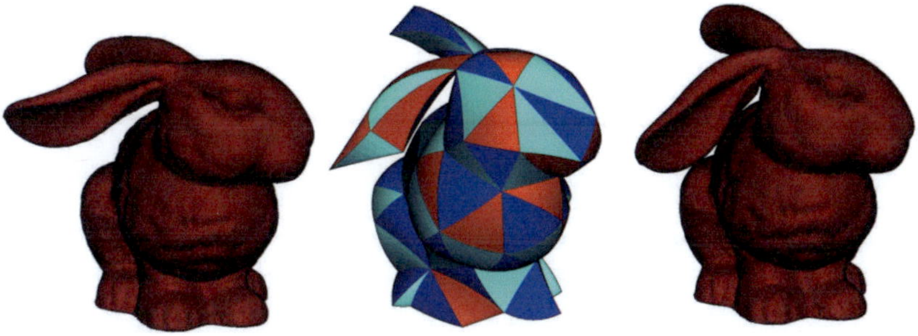

Figure 6.2.: Bunny surface mesh deforms under gravity. Volume locking is observed at ears for the simulation based on linear tetrahedra (left), while the tet10 mesh (middle) produces realistic and smooth surface deformations (right).

[Lou04]. All simulations are run on a single core of an Intel i7-930 and we use nearly incompressible material models (Poisson's ratio $\nu = 0.49$) in all scenarios.

Accuracy

The novel mapping scheme allows to accurately map high resolution surfaces to very low resolution quadratic tetrahedral grids. Fig. 6.2 shows the deformation of the Stanford Bunny under gravity. It can be seen that the surface model mapped to a quadratic mesh with 1197 DOF deforms smoothly at the ears, although the computational mesh fails to approximate the geometry in this area. In contrast, the 9468 DOF tet4 model shows severe volume locking at the ears.
The gravity induced deformation of a seahorse model is considered as a second example. We construct different low resolution computational meshes from a high resolution surface mesh with 40k triangles: A linear tetrahedral (tet4) mesh with 258 DOF and 181 elements, a linear tetrahedral mesh with 992 elements and 1488 DOF as well as a mesh with 171 quadratic elements (tet10) and 1260 DOF (see Fig. 6.3). Barycentring coordinates are used in order to map the linear tetrahedral to mesh to the high resolution surface, while the presented mapping scheme is used to embed the tet10 mesh. As was apparent from the previous simulations of

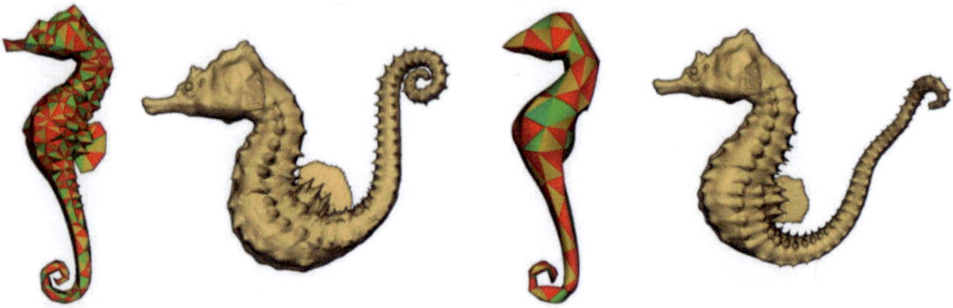

Figure 6.3.: Deformation of a seahorse model, from left to right: Linear tetrahedral FE mesh with 992 elements, the corresponding deformed surface mesh, a quadratic tetrahedral mesh with 171 elements and the deformed surface mesh mapped to the higher order FE mesh using the proposed mapping scheme.

the beam geometry, linear meshes do not deform nearly as much as the quadratic FE mesh (volume locking effect). In order to ensure visually similar deformations, we thus subject the linear meshes to higher forces in order to overcome this artificial stiffness.

For very low resolution tet4 meshes, the barycentric surface coupling results in large visible artefacts (see Fig. 6.4 left). In contrast, the proposed mapping scheme smoothly extrapolates the the deformation of the quadratic mesh is to the surface mesh and preserves local shape features. In case of the higher resolution tet4 mesh, the visible artefacts are substantially reduced. However, volumetric locking can still be observed at the end of the seahorse's tail. In contrast, the movement on the tail is much better captured by the quadratic mesh, also it has less DOF than the tet4 one (1260 vs. 1488). Furthermore, the barycentric mapping leads to a visible distortion of the seahorse's thorns even when using the higher resolution tet4 mesh (Fig. 6.4). In contrast, the novel mapping scheme preserves the shape of the thorns. The dorsal fin of the seahorse is not included in the low resolution tet10 mesh and its deformation must thus be extrapolated during the simulation. Fig. 6.4 shows that this might lead to undesirable results even if the rotation invariant mapping is employed.

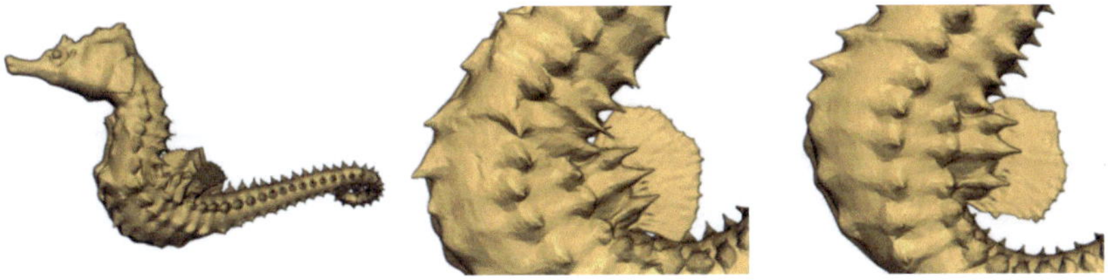

Figure 6.4.: Seahorse subjected to volumetric force: While the barycentric coupling leads to visible distortions (left, middle), the proposed mapping preserves local shape features (right).

Speed

The performance and robustness of the approach is evaluated by mapping surface and volume meshes of different resolutions. We construct two volume meshes from the Asian dragon model that is included in the Stanford 3D scanning repository with 3000 elements and 1000 elements, respectively. Furthermore, surface models with mesh size from several thousands to several 100k elements are generated. The optimization algorithms robustly finds the correct surface representation (i.e. a point $\mathbf{p}$ on the computational mesh and the corresponding distance d) for all considered surface meshes. The convergence analysis (Fig. 6.5) confirms that the numerical complexity of the algorithm is linear in the number of surface nodes and independent of the size of the coarse computational mesh.
Although the constrained Levenberg-Marquardt optimization that is run for each element is numerically complex, even large surface meshes with several 100k elements can be mapped in less than a minute thanks to the good convergence properties of the recursive scheme. Furthermore, the proposed surface representation can even be constructed in an offline process and the obtained coordinates can be simply loaded upon startup of the online simulation.

6.5.2. GPU based PCG solver

The presented FSAI based GPU solver as well as Jacobi and ILU-preconditioned approaches were implemented using the SOFA frame-

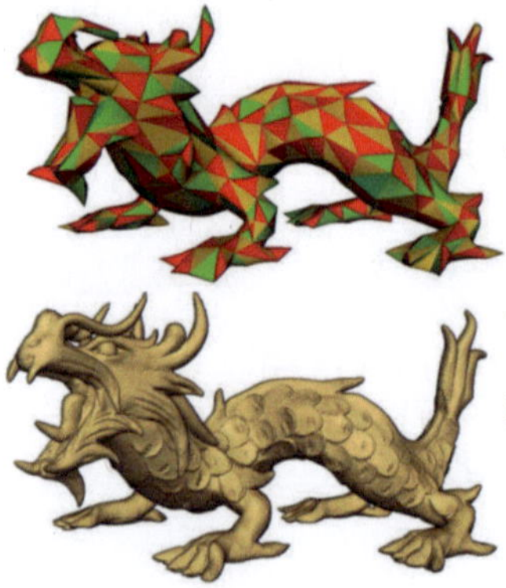

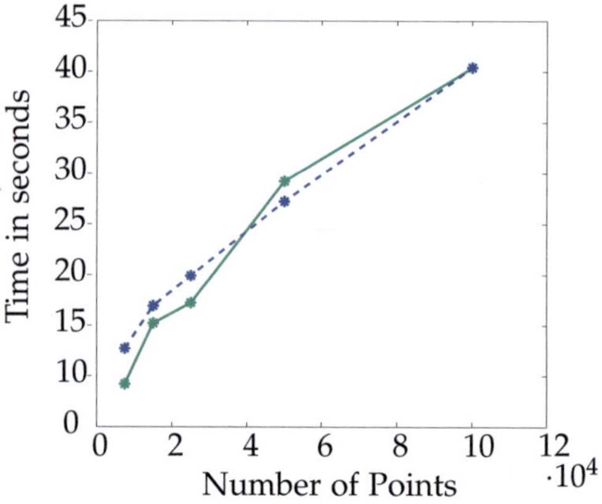

Figure 6.5.: Different surface meshes are mapped to a 3000 element mesh (blue) and a 1000 element mesh (green). The mapping time is linear in the number of points of the surface mesh and independent of the computational mesh size.

work [FDD+12] and the Paralution library. All CPU computation are performed on a single core of an Intel i7-930, while the GPU implementation is run on a Tesla C2070.

We again use the simple beam geometry under gravitational load (see Fig. 5.3) in order to assess the performance of the different solver configurations. We solve the dynamic problem with the Newmark integration method and scompute 200 time steps with a step size of $\Delta t = 0.05s$.

If the tet4 beam problem is solved using a CG-based scheme, the computation time of the nodal forces (right hand side) is negligible if compared to the linear system solve (see Fig. 6.6). For the 1461 DOF problem, the assembly of the nodal forces takes 10.39 ms on the CPU and the linear system solve is performed in 222.34 ms. Whereas for the smaller 1461 DOF problem only an acceleration factor of 1.3 is achieved by running the solver on the GPU, the large 58k DOF problem is solved more than 8 times faster on the GPU implementation. In case of the tet10 mesh, these observations are still valid, although the nodal force computations take about 10% of the total solving time in this scenario. For this reason, the GPU speed-up is a bit higher for smaller problems (1.8x for the 2217 DOF

beam). It can also be observed from Fig. 6.6 that even the GPU-based Jacobi-preconditioned CG solver is heavily outperformed by the direct single-core Pardiso solver, which solves the 1461 DOF problem in 25 ms.
As previously discussed, more complex preconditioners can speed up the CG scheme. Fig. 6.7 shows that if an ILU preconditioner is used in conjunction with the presented rotation warping scheme, a speed-up by a factor of 3.6 can be obtained. Using the highly parallelizable FSAI approach leads to a speed-up of 1.7x in comparison to the Jacobi-preconditioned algorithm. For the purpose of real-time soft tissue registration it is not necessary to compute the exact solution of the linear system for each time step. By using a residual of 0.01 as the stopping criterion for the CG iterations, a sufficient accurate solution is obtained and the solution time can be significantly reduced (Fig. 6.7 right).

6.5.3. GPU based multigrid solver

We apply the proposed GPU based multigrid (MG) scheme to the beam model under gravitational load that was presented in the previous section. We analyze a discretization with 100120 tet4 elements (57915 DOF) and a tet10-based model with 8990 elements (41781 DOF). A residual of 0.01 is used as the stopping criterion for the CG scheme. Furthermore, a grid hierarchy of 3 levels is used: For the tet4 beam the meshes consist of 100120, 8990 and 1810 elements, wheres the tet10 hierarchy is made up of meshes with 8990, 712 and 97 elements. For all MG computations, we use one iteration with a FSAI(2) scheme for smoothing purposes. The inner PCG solver uses an FSAI(2) preconditioner with rotation warping and a residual threshold of 0.01.
The results of the computations are listed in Table 6.1. For comparison purposes, we also list the corresponding timings for the direct single-core Pardiso solver and the FSAI-preconditioned GPU-CG scheme that was extensively discussed in the previous section. As the nodal forces have to be computed on all levels in order to update the elemental stiffness matrices with the current rotation, their computation time (t_{force}) is slightly higher for the MG solver. However, the additional overhead stays well below 20% for all scenarios. It is also apparent that the multigrid scheme is a very efficient preconditioner as the CG scheme only needs a few iterations to convergence. In contrast, the FSAI-PCG scheme needs

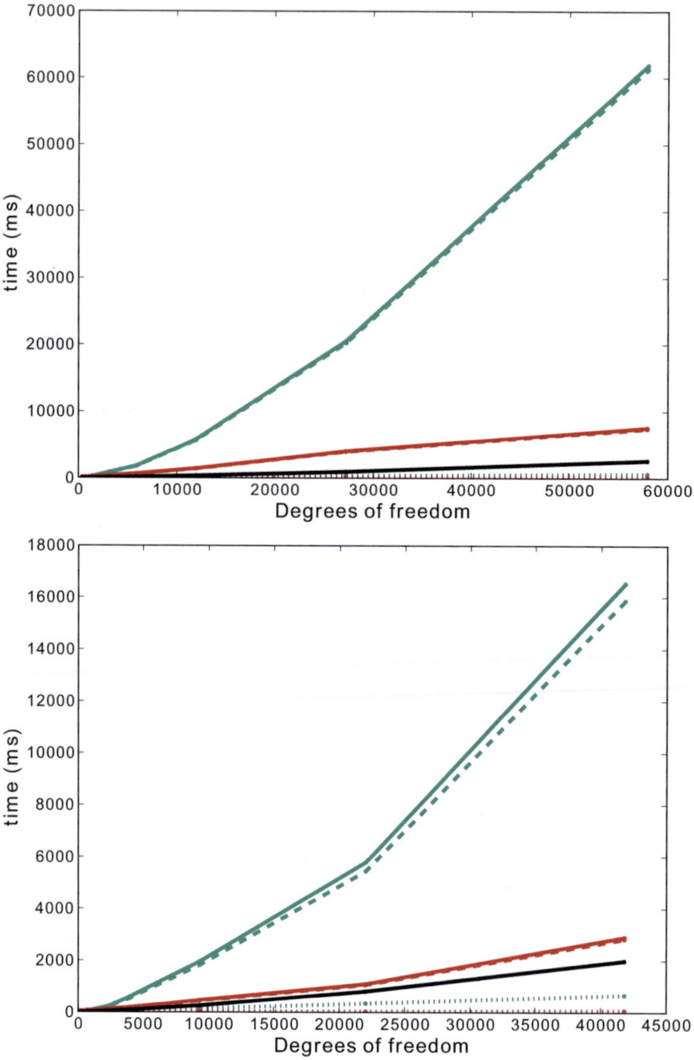

Figure 6.6.: Solution times for the tet4 beam (top) and the tet10 beam (bottom). The complete solving time per time step for a Jacobi-preconditioned CG solver on the CPU (green) and on the GPU (red) is divided into the nodal force computations (dotted line) and the linear system solve (dashed line). Total solve time for the direct solver is shown in black.

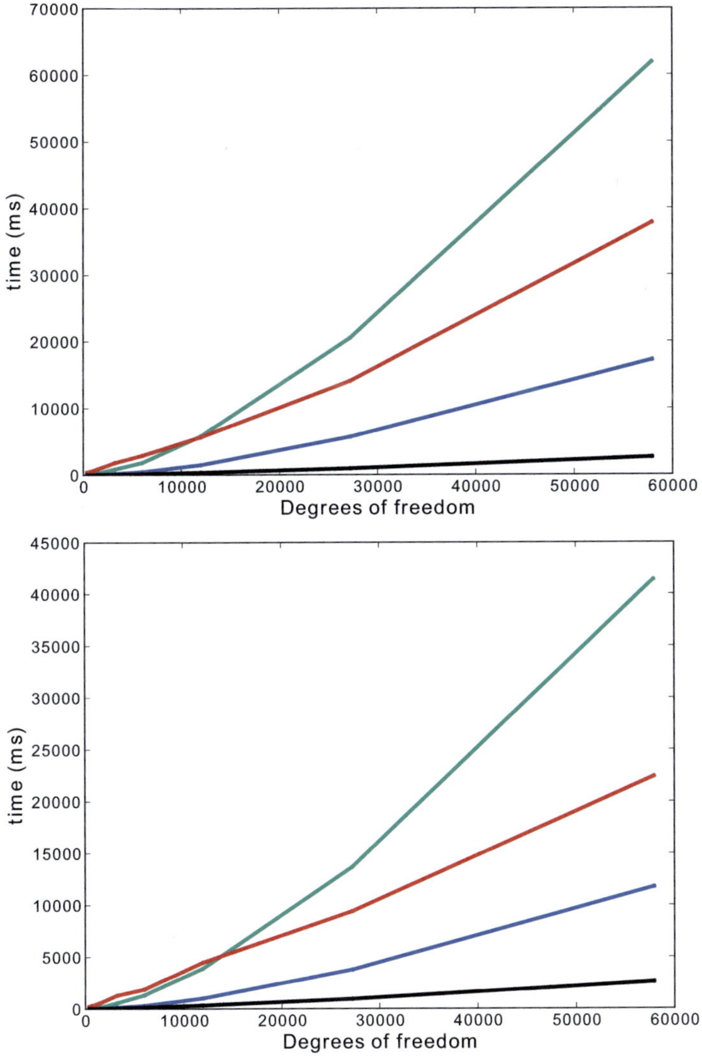

Figure 6.7.: Solution times for a CPU based CG solver scheme with a Jacobi (green), ILU (blue) and FSAI (red) preconditioner in comparison with a direct solver (black). The solution can be significantly speed up if a residual threshold of 1e-2 (bottom) is used for the CG scheme instead of computing the exact solution (top).

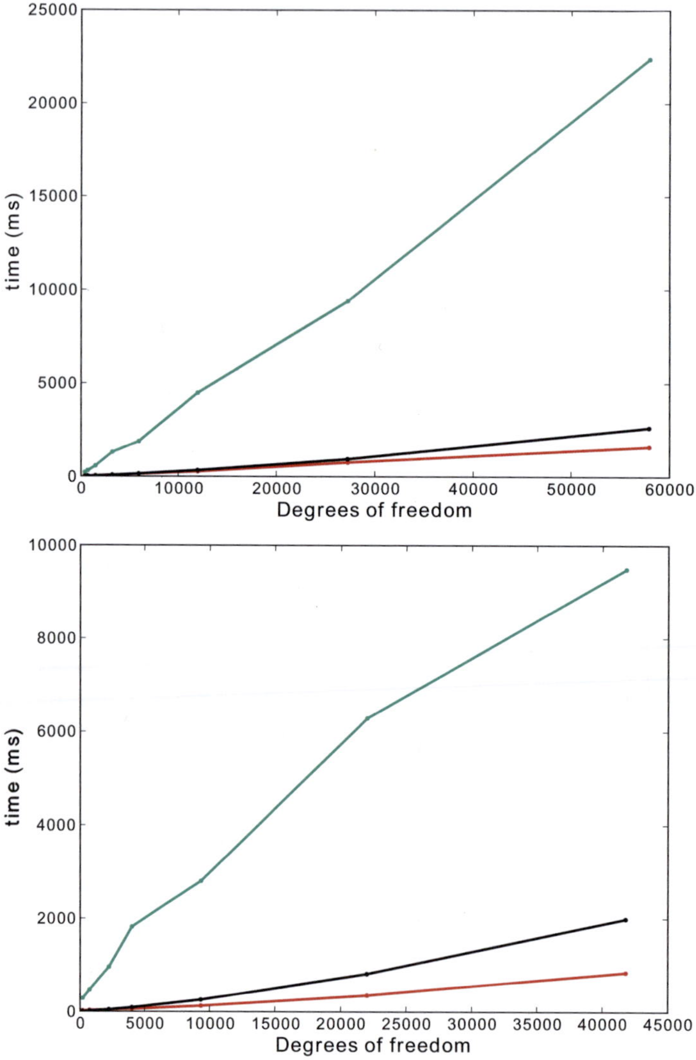

Figure 6.8.: Solution times for the tet4 beam (top) and the tet10 beam (bottom). Timings for the CPU based FSAI(2)-PCG solver (green) and the GPU variant of the algorithm (red) are listed as well as the total solve time for the direct Pardiso solver (black).

	Solver	t_{force}	t_{sm}	t_{in}	t_{pre}	t_{cg}	n_{cg}	t_{solve}	t_{tot}
tet4	Pardiso	408						2712	3120
	GPU-PCG	147			5	5	115	1314	1461
	CPU-MG	477	179	17	274	48	3	979	1476
	GPU-MG	149	20	18	54	5	3	178	327
tet10	Pardiso	621						2001	2622
	GPU-PCG	71			5	2	80	574	645
	CPU-MG	690	116	7	154	15	2	386	1076
	GPU-MG	88	22	6	35	2	2	84	172

Table 6.1.: Computation times in ms for nodal force computation t_{force}, application time for preconditioner per CG step $t_{precond}$ (for MG solvers the computation times for the smoothing operator t_{sm} and the inner solve t_{in} are listed as well) and for one pure CG step t_{cg}. Additional columns list the number of CG steps n_{cg}, the total linear solver time t_{solve} and the total computation time t_{tot} per time step in ms.

an average of 115 (tet4) and 80 (tet10) iterations. In case of the CPU variant of the MG method, the largest amount of time is spent in the smoother (179 ms per time step for the tet4 model and 116 ms for the tet10 model). This component of the algorithm can be significantly accelerated by using GPU hardware (up to 9x for the tet4 model). In contrast, the acceleration of the inner PCG solve is not as pronounced. This is due to the low size of the inner problems, which do not utilize the full computational power of the GPU.
Overall it can be seen that the proposed GPU-based multigrid scheme is a very efficient solver. For the linear tetrahedral mesh, it achieves a speed-up of nearly 10x in comparison with the direct solver (5x in comparison with the CPU-PCG approach). For the quadratic tetrahedral discretization, this difference is even more pronounced: Here, a speed-up of more than 15x is obtained in comparison with the direct solver.

6.6. Discussion

In the previous chapter we have demonstrated that quadratic tetrahedral discretizations severely outperform linear tetrahedral meshes in terms of accuracy per number of degrees of freedom. Due to volume locking, the linear tetrahedral mesh needs more than a magnitude more (up to 40x) DOF in order to achieve the same accuracy as a tet10 mesh. In this chapter, a novel mapping scheme for embedding high resolution surface models into low-resolution higher order computational meshes was proposed. The mapping is constructed using a non-linear optimization algorithm whose complexity scales linearly with the number of vertices in the surface model and is nearly independent of the number of elements in the computational model.

The main contribution of this chapter is a fast GPU-based solver for quadratic corotated FE. Based on the novel mapping scheme for higher order isoparametric meshes, a novel multigrid approach for non-conforming, unstructured grids was presented. By using a novel FSAI-preconditioned CG solver as the coarse problem solver and employing a highly parallel smoothing scheme, the developed MG solver can be efficiently implemented on the GPU. The MG scheme significantly outperforms the direct Pardiso solver as well as the state-of-the-art Jacobi-preconditioned GPU-CG solver by more than an order of magnitude. It allows to simulate a high resolution, 8990 tet10 elements (41781 DOF) problem at nearly 6 time steps per second. As we will see in the upcoming chapter, this model size definitely provides sufficient accuracy in order to be used in a soft tissue registration scheme.

All things are difficult before they are easy.
— Thomas Fuller

7.

Physics based shape matching

In the last chapters we concluded that corotated finite elements offer an efficient, yet accurate way to model the mechanical response of soft tissue for registration purposes (chapter 5). We also learned how these models can be efficiently solved on the GPU (chapter 6). In this chapter, we present a novel method for imposing the intraoperative sensor data as boundary conditions on the biomechanical model in order to perform an accurate registration. As detailed in chapter 3, we in particular deal with two kinds of scenarios. First, we match a given intraoperative partial surface of an organ to a preoperative biomechanical model. This set-up can be used in order to determine an initial non-rigid registration. Furthermore, we show how known landmark displacements from endoscopic images or US tracking can be incorporated in the formulation.
We describe non-rigid surface registration as an electrostatic-elastic problem, where an elastic body that is electrically charged (preoperative model) slides into an oppositely charged rigid shape (intraoperative surface). Consequently, we call this approach physics based shape matching (PBSM). The elastic energy of the deformed organ is described by a finite element based biomechanical model, while the correspondence is enforced by the electrostatic field. As the technique is based on a preoperative volumetric FE model, it naturally recovers the position of volumetric structures (e.g. tumors or vessels).
The novel physics based interpretation allows casting the shape matching problem into a single variational formulation. We show how this approach can be used for robust parameter control, partial surface matching and the integration of landmark correspondences. In addition to the unified mathematical formulation, key contributions in comparison with related work are the use of a more accurate non-linear model (compared

with [CMS+05] [DCDM10] [RWC+13]) and the ability to match partial surfaces (compared with [CPC+07] [BSD+05]). Furthermore, PBSM can achieve near real-time performance and can be combined with landmark based approaches (e.g. texture tracking). The method is not only evaluated through extensive simulations studies, but we also demonstrate in a phantom experiment how liver models can be registered from stereo endoscopic data.

In the following section the variational formulation of the electrostatic-elastic problem and its discretization using the FEM is presented. Furthermore, we outline a physics based stabilization technique and describe adaptive control mechanisms for the PBMS parameters. Additionally, an extension of the scheme for partial surface matching is proposed. We present a detailed evaluation of the method using *in silico* test data on three liver surface models. Furthermore, we show by means of a phantom experiment how the PBSM scheme can be used to match a preoperative liver model to an intraoperative surface model that has been acquired using stereo endoscopic images.

7.1. Variational formulation

7.1.1. Electric potential induced by the deformed surface

Full electrostatic formulation

The deformed intraoperative surface is modeled as a rigid shape that has a uniformly distributed surface charge. In order to derive the electric potential that is induced by the charge, we create an unstructured tetrahedral volume mesh in a sufficiently large area around the surface. We then discretize Laplace's equation

$$\Delta\phi = 0 \qquad \phi = \overline{\phi} \text{ on } \partial\Omega \tag{7.1}$$

on this grid using the finite element method. All nodes on the deformed surface are assigned a zero potential, while all nodes on the boundary of the box volume are assigned their distance to the surface. Upon solving the discretized problem, each node J in the volume mesh is assigned a potential value $\boldsymbol{\phi}_J$. The potential at an arbitrary sample point $\mathbf{s}_\mathcal{T}$ can be computed by first finding the element $\mathcal{E}$ in which the point is located before calculating the associated local coordinates ξ_s in $\mathcal{E}$. The potential ϕ and the potential gradient $\nabla\phi$ at s are then given by the linear combinations

$$\phi(\mathbf{s}_\mathcal{T}) = \boldsymbol{\phi}_J N_J(\xi_s) \quad \text{and} \quad \nabla\phi(\mathbf{s}_\mathcal{T}) = \boldsymbol{\phi}_J \nabla N_J(\xi_s) \tag{7.2}$$

of $\boldsymbol{\phi}_J$ weighted with the the 4 basis functions N_J (or the gradient of the basis functions ∇N_J) evaluated at ξ_s.

Distance field approximation

Although the FEM-based solution of Laplace's equation allows an accurate computation of the electric potential field, the approach is computationally intensive. First of all, an unstructured tetrahedral volume mesh has to be intraoperatively generated for each deformed surface. Furthermore, the sampling of the potential field stored as an unstructured grid is a bottleneck of the algorithm. In order to overcome both problems, the electric potential can be approximated by a distance field. In this case, the potential values can be sampled using a collision detection scheme during the simulation. A numerical finite difference scheme with a reasonably large sample distance has to be used in order to compute the potential gradient. In order to minimize the number of necessary samples, we restrict the linearization to the forces that act in the direction of the surface normal and compute the associated gradient

$$\nabla\phi(\mathbf{s}_\mathcal{T}) \approx \frac{\partial\phi(\mathbf{s}_\mathcal{T})}{\partial\mathbf{n}}\mathbf{n}, \quad \frac{\partial\phi(\mathbf{s}_\mathcal{T})}{\partial\mathbf{n}} \approx \frac{\phi(\mathbf{s}_\mathcal{T} + \frac{1}{2}h\mathbf{n}) - \phi(\mathbf{s}_\mathcal{T} - \frac{1}{2}h\mathbf{n})}{h} \tag{7.3}$$

by calculating the 1D derivative $\partial\phi/\partial\mathbf{n}$ using a finite difference scheme with sampling distance h.

7.1.2. Variational formulation of the electrostatic-elastic problem

The registration problem is solved by finding a deformation $\varphi : \mathbf{X} \mapsto \mathbf{x}$ that maps each material point $\mathbf{X}$ in the initial configuration Ω_0 to the point $\mathbf{x}$ in the deformed configuration Ω such that Ω approximates the given shape. We use the described corotated elasticity model to model the internal elastic energy I_{int} in terms of the corotated Cauchy stress tensor σ^{CR} and the corotated Cauchy strain tensor ϵ^{CR}. Furthermore, we assign a uniform surface charge with density q to the boundary $\partial\Omega$ of the elastic body. Thus, the total energy of the electrostatic-elastic system

$$\mathrm{I} = \mathrm{I}_{int} + \mathrm{I}_{\Phi} = \int_{\Omega} \frac{1}{2}\sigma^{CR} : \epsilon^{CR} \mathrm{dV} + \int_{\partial\Omega} q\phi \mathrm{dA} \tag{7.4}$$

can be expressed as the sum of the internal elastic energy I_{int} and the electrostatic potential energy I_{Φ}. We now seek a deformation mapping φ that is a stationary point of I, i.e.

$$< \delta\mathrm{I}[\mathbf{x}], \delta\mathbf{x} > \stackrel{!}{=} 0. \tag{7.5}$$

For the derivation of the variational form

$$< \delta\mathrm{I}_{int}[\mathbf{x}], \delta\mathbf{x} > = \int_{\Omega} \frac{1}{2}\sigma^{CR} : \delta\epsilon^{CR} \mathrm{dV} \tag{7.6}$$

of the internal elastic energy we refer to chapter 5. We also point out that the formulation can easily be reduced to a linear elastic approach by simply inserting the linear stress and strain measures (i.e. σ, ϵ). In order to express the variation of the electrical potential energy $\phi(\mathbf{x})$, we use the Hessian $H^{\phi}(\mathbf{x}_t)$ to develop the electric potential into the Taylor series

$$\phi(\mathbf{x}) \approx \phi(\mathbf{x}_t) + (\mathbf{x} - \mathbf{x}_t)\nabla\phi(\mathbf{x}_t) + \frac{1}{2}(\mathbf{x} - \mathbf{x}_t)^T H^{\phi}(\mathbf{x}_t)(\mathbf{x} - \mathbf{x}_t) \tag{7.7}$$

around $\mathbf{x}_t$. The variational form is then given by

$$\begin{aligned} < \delta\mathrm{I}_{pot}[\mathbf{x}], \delta\mathbf{x} > &= \int_{\partial\Omega} \frac{\mathrm{d}}{\mathrm{dh}}(\phi(\mathbf{x} + h\delta\mathbf{x})q\mathrm{dA}\Big|_{h=0} \\ &= \int_{\partial\Omega} \left(\delta\mathbf{x}\nabla\phi + \delta\mathbf{x}H^{\phi}(\mathbf{x}_t)(\mathbf{x} - \mathbf{x}_t)\right) q\mathrm{dA}. \end{aligned} \tag{7.8}$$

Until now we have expressed the energy densities with reference to the (unknown) deformed configuration. We now seek to formulate the variational form in terms of the initial configuration. First, we introduce the initial surface charge density q_0 on the undeformed infinitesimal surface element dA_0 and assume that the surface charge is conserved, i.e. $q dA = q_0 dA_0$. Furthermore, we follow the standard linear elasticity approximation and just replace the integral in eq. (7.6) over Ω with the integral over Ω_0 without performing a Piola transform [BLM00]. Thus, we obtain the continuous variational form

$$\int_{\Omega_0} \frac{1}{2}\sigma^{CR} : \delta\epsilon^{CR} dV_0 + \int_{\partial\Omega_0} \left(\nabla\phi + H^{\phi}(\mathbf{x}_t)(\mathbf{x}-\mathbf{x}_t)\right)\delta\mathbf{x} q_0 dA_0 = 0 \quad (7.9)$$

that describes the registration problem.

7.2. Discretization and algorithm design

7.2.1. Discrete formulation

We construct a finite element approximation for φ on a linear tetrahedral mesh. Thus, within each element the deformation field $\mathbf{x}$ is expressed by $\mathbf{x} = \mathcal{X}_{jJ} N_J$. Here, the entries of the vector $\mathcal{X}_{jJ}$ describe the position of the J-th node in the spatial direction j in the deformed configuration. In FE theory for elasticity, the internal nodal forces in the direction i at node I are accumulated in the discrete force vector $\mathbf{f}^{int} = f^{int}_{iI}$. Similarly, we define the vector $\mathbf{f}^{\phi}$ that contains the electric forces that are induced by the potential field. We use a FE Galerkin approach and approximate the surface integral in eq. (7.9) over each surface triangle with the one-point Gaussian quadrature at sample point $\mathbf{s}_{\mathcal{T}}$ with the local coordinates ξ_s. The force at each node for a given deformation $\mathbf{x}$

$$\mathbf{f}^{\phi}(\mathbf{x}) = f^{\phi}_{iI}(\mathbf{x}) = \frac{1}{2} q_0 A_{\mathcal{T}} \nabla\phi(\mathbf{s}_{\mathcal{T}})_i N_I(\xi_s) \qquad \text{and} \qquad s_{\mathcal{T}} = \mathcal{X}_{jJ} N_J(\xi_s) \quad (7.10)$$

are then calculated by summing the contributions of each surface triangle $\mathcal{T}$ with area $A_{\mathcal{T}}$ around the node. As described in section 7.1.1, the potential field gradient $\nabla\phi(\mathbf{s}_{\mathcal{T}})$ is sampled from the unstructured grid data structure if a Laplacian potential field is used, while it is computed from potential field samples if the distance field approximation is employed. Using the obtained nodal force vectors, the discretized form of equation 7.9 reads

$$\mathbf{f}^{int}(\mathbf{x}) + \mathbf{f}^{\phi}(\mathbf{x}) = 0. \quad (7.11)$$

In order to solve this highly non-linear equation, the forces have to be linearized with respect to the nodal displacements. In analogy to the elastic global stiffness matrix $\mathbf{K}^{int} = \partial \mathbf{f}^{int} / \partial \mathcal{X}$ [BLM00] we define the global tangent electrostatic stiffness matrix $\mathbf{K}^{\phi} = \partial \mathbf{f}^{\phi} / \partial \mathcal{X}$. The linearization of eq. (7.11) around ${}^{t}\mathbf{x}$ is then given by

$$(\mathbf{K}^{\phi} + \mathbf{K}^{int})\mathrm{d}\chi = \mathbf{K}\mathrm{d}\chi = -\mathbf{f}^{\phi}({}^{t}\mathbf{x}) - \mathbf{f}^{int}({}^{t}\mathbf{x}). \tag{7.12}$$

with the displacement vector $\mathrm{d}\chi = \mathcal{X} - {}^{t}\mathcal{X}$. Similar to the nodal force calculations (7.10), the 12x12 elemental electrostatic stiffness matrix for tetrahedron $\mathcal{E}$

$$\mathbf{K}^{\phi,\mathcal{E}}_{iIjJ} = \frac{1}{2} q_0 A_{\mathcal{T}} H^{\phi}_{ij}(\mathbf{s}_{\mathcal{T}}) N_I(\xi_s) N_J(\xi_s) \tag{7.13}$$

is calculated by sampling the contributions of each surface triangle $\mathcal{T}$ in $\mathcal{E}$. The evaluation of the Hessian $H^{\phi}(\mathbf{s}_{\mathcal{T}})$ has to be performed numerically for both the Laplacian potential and the distance field approximation. Here, we again restrict the linearization to the forces that act in the direction of the surface normal and compute the associated Hessian

$$H^{\phi}_{ij}(\mathbf{s}_{\mathcal{T}}) \approx \frac{\partial^2 \phi(\mathbf{s}_{\mathcal{T}})}{\partial \mathbf{n}^2} (n_i \otimes n_j), \tag{7.14}$$

$$\frac{\partial^2 \phi(\mathbf{s}_{\mathcal{T}})}{\partial \mathbf{n}^2} \approx \frac{\phi(\mathbf{s}_{\mathcal{T}} + h \cdot \mathbf{n}) - 2\phi(\mathbf{s}_{\mathcal{T}}) + \phi(\mathbf{s}_{\mathcal{T}} - h \cdot \mathbf{n})}{h^2} \tag{7.15}$$

by using a second order central difference scheme.

7.2.2. Dynamic registration scheme

A straight forward successive solution of the linearized problem in a Newton-Raphson scheme is numerically unstable for most registration problems, because of the strong non-linearities in the original problem (7.11). We introduce a physics based stabilization scheme by not just considering the static linearized equilibrium (7.12), but instead modeling the dynamics of the system. For this purpose we model the viscoelastic effects with Rayleigh damping. Thus, we introduce the mass matrix $\mathbf{M}$ and the damping matrix $\mathbf{C} = \alpha\mathbf{M} + \beta\mathbf{K}$ in order to obtain

$$\mathbf{M}\mathrm{d}\ddot{\chi} + \mathbf{D}\mathrm{d}\dot{\chi} + \mathbf{K}\mathrm{d}\chi = -\mathbf{f}^{\phi}({}^{t}\mathbf{x}) - \mathbf{f}^{int}({}^{t}\mathbf{x}). \tag{7.16}$$

The system of ordinary differential equations (7.16) is solved using the constant-average-acceleration scheme of the β-Newmark method (see section 5.3.2).

7.2.3. Adaptive parameter control

For most non-rigid registration algorithms, the main parameter of the method is the ratio between the internal regularization energy and the external energy that drives the deformation. In the PBSM approach this is represented by the surface charge density q_0 and the elastic modulus E. During the registration process we control q_0 based on a simple energy criterion. Starting from a very small charge $q_0(t_0)$, we update the q_0 for each time step by comparing the total elastic energy I_{int} and the total potential energy I_Φ:

$$q_0(t+1) = q_0(t)\mathrm{I}_{int}/\mathrm{I}_\Phi \tag{7.17}$$

If the sampling distance h for the gradient and Hessian computation is too low or too high, the method can become unstable. However, the parameter can be varied over a large range without affecting the stability or the accuracy of the method: For all examples that we analyzed the PBSM scheme converges for sampling distance from 2 mm to 20 mm.
All other problem-specific parameters (i.e. the density ρ, elastic parameters λ, μ and viscoelastic parameters α, β) are directly given by the physical properties of the organ. It has to be pointed out that the method is very robust to variations of these parameters. Furthermore we noticed that the convergence speed can be slightly increased if the viscoelastic damping is minimally more pronounced than the real viscoelastic behavior of soft tissue ($\alpha = 0.6$, $\beta = 0.2$).

7.2.4. Integration of known landmark correspondences

In some intraoperative scenarios, a sparse set of landmark correspondences is available. In the context of initial registration, these can be imprecise surface landmarks obtained from manual input or automatically computed surface features. Furthermore, texture tracking can be used for continuous real-time registration during the intervention. If intraoperative US is available, it is even possible to determine a limited

number of volumetric landmark correspondences (e.g. vessel bifurcations).
A straightforward approach is to use these correspondences to compute an initial rigid alignment. As the iterative linearization of the energy functional can be regarded as an ICP-like scheme for non-rigid registration, it is intuitively clear that the PBSM approach inherits many convergence properties of the iterative closest point (ICP) algorithm. Thus, a poor initial alignment which involves strong rotations prevents the method from finding the correct correspondences as it becomes trapped in a local minimum. The convergence of the PBSM method can be ensured by performing an initial rigid alignment based on landmark correspondences ahead of the core algorithm. This can be done in an automatic, robust way using shape-descriptor based methods [dSGF+12] [dSSK+14].
If precise landmark correspondences are available, it might be more desirable to directly integrate these deformation constraints into the variational formulation eq. (7.9). A straightforward way to do this is to impose the known correspondences as displacement constraints. However, noise and outliers in the sensor data can lead to large artefacts that might even impair the stability of the method. Therefore, we impose the constraints in a weaker way using Robin boundary conditions. Physically, this can be interpreted as connecting the landmarks through stiff springs. Here, the problem arises that the landmarks' positions do usually not coincide with the node positions of the finite element mesh. In order to overcome this problem we compute the barycentric coordinates for each landmark with respect to the nearest element. Subsequently, we use the barycentric proportions to divide the spring forces among the element's nodes.

7.2.5. Matching of partial surfaces

In the intraoperative setting, organ surfaces are only partially visible. In this scenario, there are surfaces where the displacement is not known and that cannot be matched to the known partial surface. In order to accommodate these requirements, the PBSM scheme has to be adapted. During the matching, only those surface areas have to be activated (i.e. given an electrical surface charge) that do indeed correspond to the known partial surface. We use two simple geometric criteria to select active triangles: First, we demand that the triangle has to be sufficiently

close to the deformed (intraoperative) surface mesh. In addition, the current normal of a triangle in the deforming volume model must be similar to the normal of the corresponding triangle in the deformed surface mesh in order for the triangle to be activated.
This approach works well for structures that are close to the known partial surface. However, the registration accuracy of structures on the far side of the organ can suffer. Furthermore, the registration can even break down if the partial surface is too small. One way to overcome this problem is to use additional landmarks and integrate them as described in the previous section. Similarly, a-priori information about the movement of organ surfaces can be imposed. For example, areas with negligible motion can be fixed during the registration process (see e.g. [HDB+13]). A different path can be taken if landmarks inside the organ are known (e.g. through ultrasound). Then, an optimization scheme on top of the PBSM approach can be used in order to resolve the movements of the hidden surfaces (similar to the work of Alterovitz et al. [AGP+06] and Ruckert et al. [RWC+13]).

7.3. Accuracy and performance validation

The PBSM algorithm was implemented using the SOFA framework [FDD+12]. All simulations were run on a single core of an Intel i7-930 CPU using the direct PARDISO linear solver from the Intel MKL. We used a time step of 0.5s and the viscoelastic parameters of $\alpha = 0.6, \beta = 0.2$ for all scenarios.

7.3.1. In silico evaluation

High resolution FE models were constructed from three different segmented liver datasets. In order to establish a ground truth deformation, we subsequently applied a respiratory deformation pattern to these models using the ABAQUS FEM package and a hyperelastic Neo-Hookean material model (see Fig. 7.1). For each scenario, the surface mesh of the undeformed and the deformed liver were extracted in order to serve as the input for the shape matching. Furthermore, partial surface meshes were selected that contain approx. half of the complete deformed surface. Finally, we generated low resolution tetrahedral meshes elements for

	DOF ground truth	max disp. [mm]	mean disp. [mm]	DOF PBSM model
Liver #1	48873	35.03	9.97	6147
Liver #2	49920	29.22	7.46	6096
Liver #3	79158	56.68	9.17	6285

Table 7.1.: Size of the ground truth model in terms of DOF, maximal displacement (max disp.) and mean displacement (mean disp.) as well as size of the PBSM model for the three livers considered in the *in silico* study.

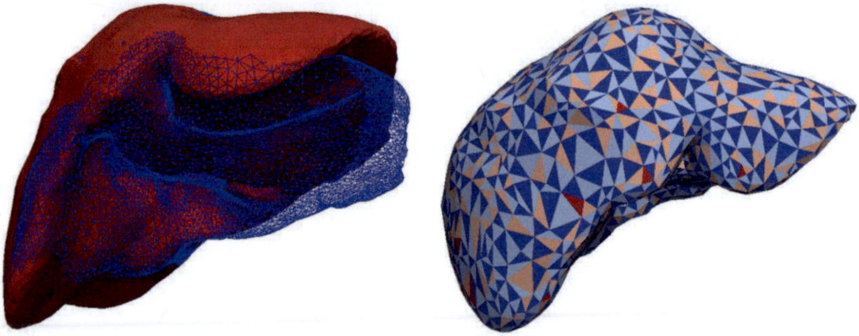

Figure 7.1.: Left: Undeformed liver (red) is matched to a deformed surface (blue). Right: Lower resolution FE model used to run the PBSM scheme.

the PBSM scheme. Model sizes in terms of degrees of freedom (DOF) and quantitative details on the imposed deformation are given in Table. 7.1.

Accuracy

The accuracy of the distance field based algorithm (DF-PBSM) is compared to the approach based on the Laplacian potential field (LP-PBSM) (see Fig. 7.2). For this comparison, a linear FE model is used for regularization. The error is measured by obtaining the Euclidean distance of the computed deformation at each point of the ground truth mesh. For

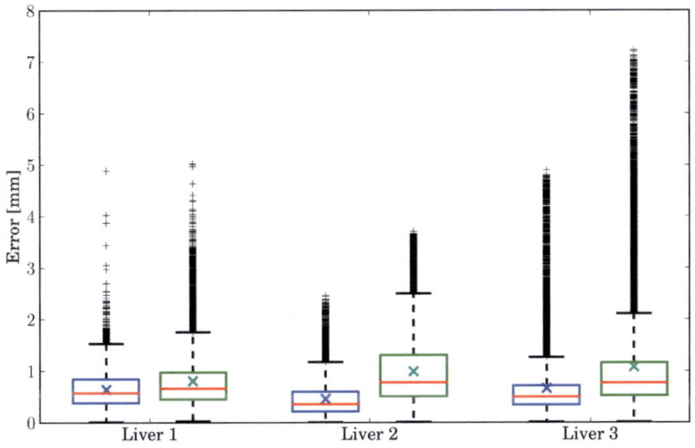

Figure 7.2.: Error distribution of the distance field based based approach (blue) and the Laplacian potential field based PBSM (green). The mean is denoted by the red line, while averages are shown using crosses.

this purpose the ground truth mesh is mapped to the lower resolution PBSM mesh using barycentric mapping. Mean error values for DF-PBSM (0.64 mm, 0.46 mm and 0.66 mm) are significantly lower than for the scheme based on the Laplacian field (0.8 mm, 0.99 mm and 1.08 mm) in all three scenarios. This can be attributed to the fact that the resolution of the FE grid which is used for the potential field computation is not high enough to fully capture the geometry of the deformed surface. In contrast the distance sampling is performed on the high resolution deformed surface.

In a second study we analyzed the impact of the non-linear elasticity model. Fig. 7.3 shows that the mean error values for the three scenarios (0.43 mm, 0.32 mm, 0.46 mm) are clearly reduced in comparison with the linear elasticity model. When comparing the volume errors (blue) and the surface errors (green) it becomes apparent that the highest errors occurr at the surface of the models.

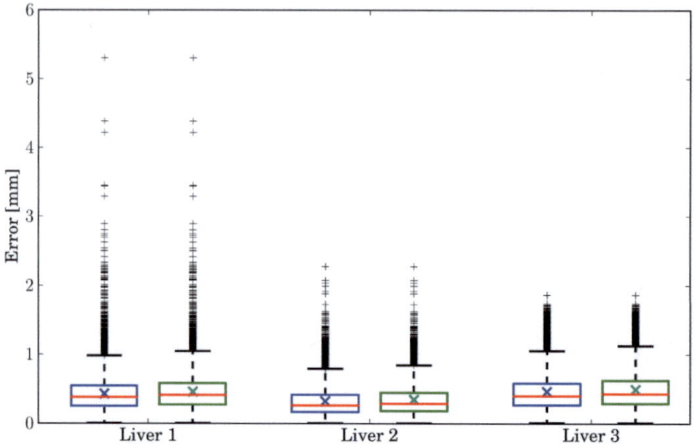

Figure 7.3.: Volumetric (blue) and surface (green) error distribution for the PBSM matching using a non-linear elastic model. The mean is denoted by the red line, while averages are shown using crosses.

The geometric distribution of the surface error for the first liver scenario is displayed in Fig. 7.4: While the overall error remains well below 2 mm, error spikes can be observed on the bottom of the liver. In this area, the lower resolution computational mesh cannot capture all details of the ground truth mesh. Similar error patterns can be observed for the other example models. One possibility to reduce these errors is to use higher resolution models for the PBSM scheme.

In a follow-up study we compare the accuracy of the non-linear DF-PBSM scheme to the coherent point drift (CPD) algorithm. This state-of-the-art method treat the registration process as a probability density estimation problem and uses a regularization term that ensures the smoothness of the deformation [MS10]. In contrast to the PBSM scheme, the CPD approach does not use a volumetric model. Therefore, only surface displacements can be compared and it is not possible to map the ground truth mesh to the test model using barycentric mapping. We thus interpolate the ground truth displacements to all nodes of the lower resolution surface test model and measure the Euclidean distance at each

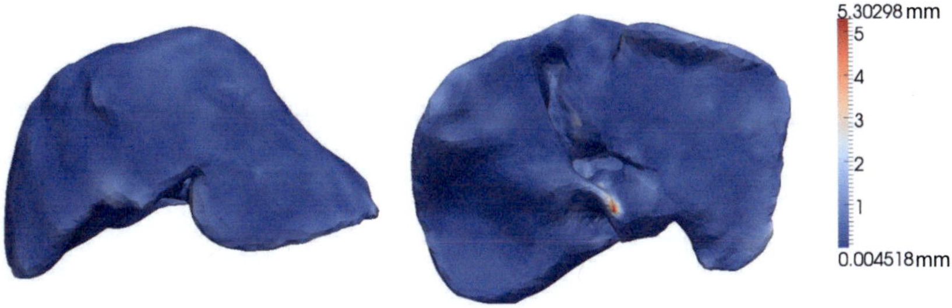

Figure 7.4.: Geometrical error distribution of the liver #1 model when matched using non-linear elastic regularization.

of these nodes. The mean error values of the PBSM method (0.49 mm, 0.33 mm, 0.49 mm) are much lower than the CPD mean error (1.96 mm, 3.22 mm, 3.95 mm). It is apparent from Fig. 7.5 that the same pattern can be observed for the average and maximum error. Fig. 7.6 shows while PBSM clearly outperforms CPD in terms of accuracy: Whereas the CPD scheme ensures that all points are close to the surface, large tangential displacement errors occur. This is especially true in areas that exhibit very few surface features. In contrast, the much better biomechanical based regularization of PBSM ensures a high accuracy even in these regions.
In the intraoperative setting, typically only partial surfaces are available. In order to mimic this setting, partial surfaces that cover approx. half of the complete deformed surface were obtained. The preoperative volume model is subsequently matched to the partial surface using DF-PBSM and the corotated elasticity model. Naturally, the registration error is much higher in those areas that are not covered by the partial surface (see Fig. 7.7). This is reflected in the mean errors (1.97 mm, 1.69 mm and 2.24 mm) and the error distributions (Fig. 7.8). However, the registration accuracy is high in those areas covered by the partial surface (Fig. 7.7). In a typical surgical setting this is usually the most important area. One possibility to increase the registration accuracy in areas away from the partial surface is to use US imaging to find additional landmark correspondences. In the *in silico* study we added a correspondence at the point with the highest error. This clearly improves the overall registration accuracy (Fig. 7.7, 7.8).

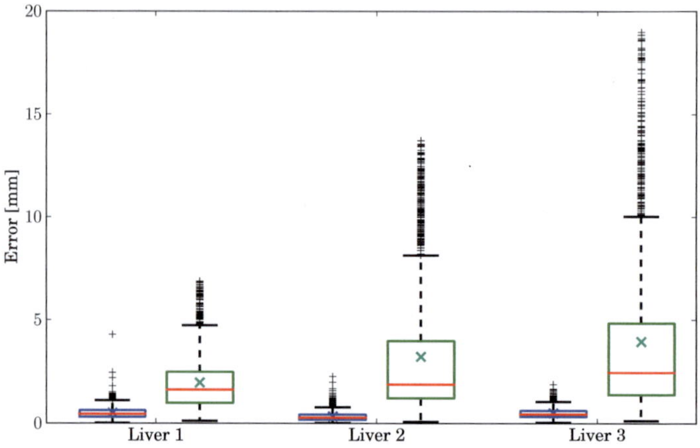

Figure 7.5.: PBSM (blue) vs. CPD (green) error distribution. The mean is denoted by the red line, while averages are shown using crosses.

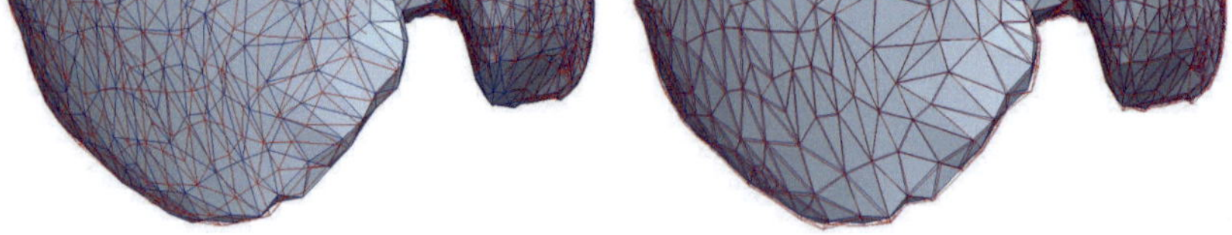

Figure 7.6.: Ground truth solution (light blue and blue wireframe) is compared to the CPD-based registration (left, red wireframe) as well as the PBSM-based registration (right, red wireframe).

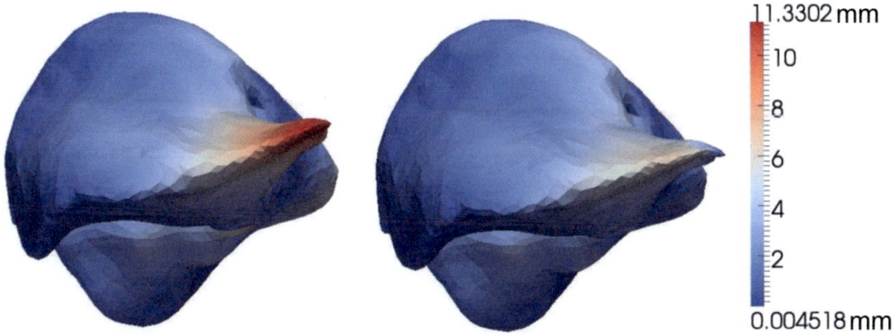

Figure 7.7.: The left part of the liver not covered by the partial surface exhibits much higher registration errors (left). These errors can be significantly reduced if an additional landmark correspondence is known (green).

Stability and Speed

It has already been discussed that the method can get trapped in local minima if the initial alignment is very poor. In order to overcome this problem we use a shape-descriptor based rigid registration algorithm [dSGF$^+$12] ahead of the non-rigid PBSM iterations (Fig. 7.9). With this configuration, we observed convergence for all scenarios.
In order to assess the performance of the DF-PBSM method, we monitored the number of iterations until the maximum error was within 0.1 mm of the final error and the number of time steps per second (TPS). As can be seen from Table. 7.2, the total registration time ranges from 7s to 19s. It should be noted that all computations were performed using an unoptimized, single core implementation of the PBSM method. The current bottleneck of the algorithm is the sampling of the electrostatic surface forces using a collision detection scheme. This is an inherently parallel problem and it is very well suited for multi-core and massively parallel platforms. We also note that the algorithm performs around 2 time steps per second for the chosen problem sizes. This is important as an optimized version can process intraoperative sensor data (e.g. landmark positions from texture tracking) in real-time.

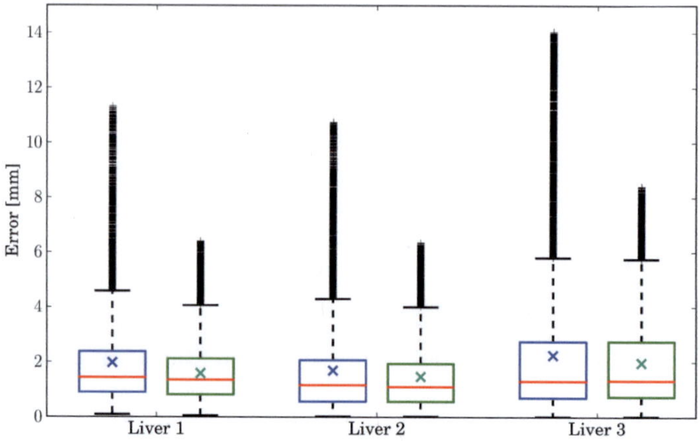

Figure 7.8.: Error distribution for the PBSM matching using a non-linear elastic model and partial surfaces (blue). These errors can be significantly reduced if an additional landmark correspondence is known (green). The mean is denoted by the red line, while averages are shown using crosses.

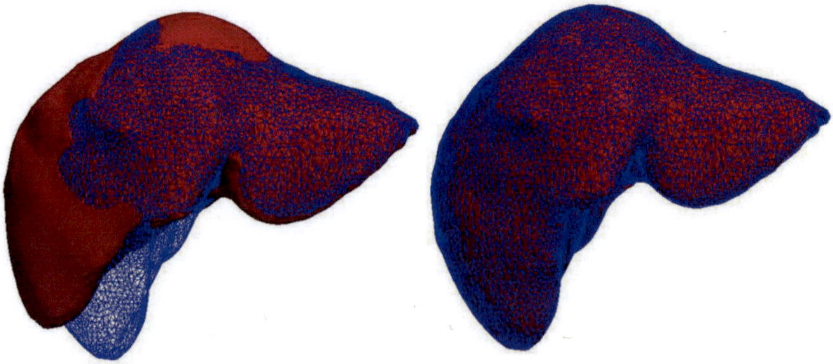

Figure 7.9.: If an initial rigid alignement is performed (left), the PBSM scene converges for all scenarios (right).

	DOF	iterations	TPS	time (s)
Liver #1	6147	22	1.99	11.06
Liver #2	6096	15	2.12	7.08
Liver #3	6285	36	1.94	18.56

Table 7.2.: Model size, iteration count, timesteps per second (TPS) and total registration time for the analyzed liver models.

7.3.2. Phantom experiment

We performed an indentation on a silicon phantom (see Fig. 7.10). The ground truth is obtained by tracking the displacement of 6 small teflon marker balls in CT scans of the phantom (see Fig. 7.10). A volumetric mesh of the undeformed phantom is constructed from segmented CT data. We then use PBSM to map three different surface meshes to the volumetric mesh (Fig. 7.11): 1. A complete surface mesh of the deformed phantom obtained from segmented CT data. 2. A partial surface obtained from segmented CT images 3. A partial surface obtained from stereo endoscopic images. The surface was obtained using dense 3D reconstruction [RBS+12], random-forest based segmentation of the liver and image stitching. In line with related work [CMS+05] [HDP+13] we fix small parts of the liver that have negligible motion (see Fig. 7.11) for all partial surface matchings.
The maximal displacement of the tracked marker balls is 46.6 mm with a mean displacement of 23.9 mm. The PBMS scheme remains stable and converges to a solution for all scenarios. The mean error for the complete surface matching (scenario 1) is 2.6 mm (max. error 4.9 mm). Several factors contribute to the significantly larger errors in the phantom experiment than in the *in silico* evaluations: First of all the ground truth data can be inaccurate due to errors during the segmentation process. Furthermore, the strong indentation (Fig. 7.10) in the experiment leads to large variations near the indenter. Fig. 7.10 also reveals that the error increases for partial surface matching (mean error of 4.96 mm). In a similar pattern that has been observed during the *in silico* experiments this is mainly caused by the markers that lie away from the partial surface.

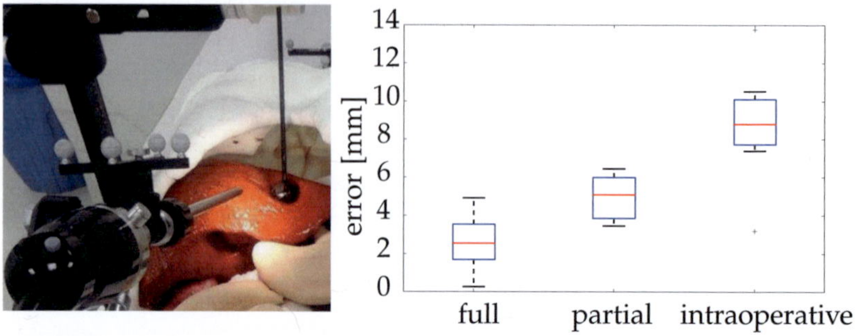

Figure 7.10.: Indentation on a liver phantom: Experimental setup (left) and error distribution in case the full CT-reconstructed surface, a partial CT-surface or the intraoperative surface is used (right).

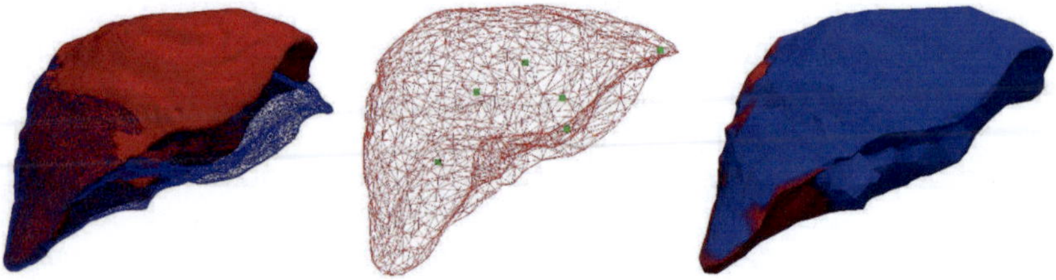

Figure 7.11.: Matching of a complete surface (left), position of markers inside the liver phantom (middle) and fixed nodes on the liver marked in red (right).

Although the matching to the intraoperatively acquired surface (scenario 3) gives visually satisfactory results, the error is rather high (mean error 8.7 mm). In addition to errors that occur during surface acquisition, this can be mainly attributed to the fact that the acquired surface is too small to adequately capture the deformation.

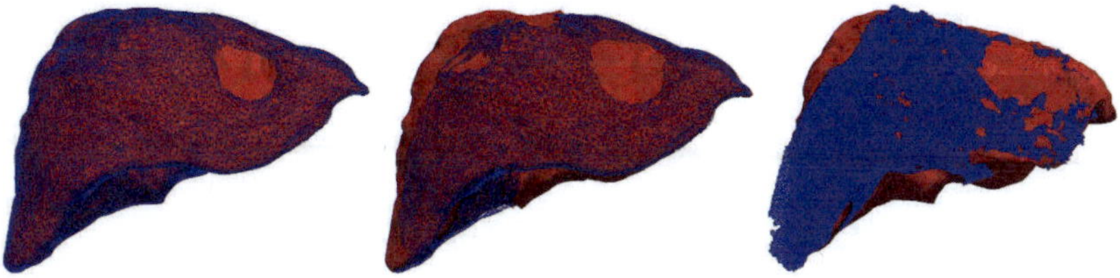

Figure 7.12.: Matching of a complete surface (left), a partial surface obtained from CT images (middle) and matching of an intra-operatively acquired surface (right).

7.4. Discussion

The novel PBMS approach allows a robust, landmark-free registration of multi-modal surfaces for image guided surgery. It is robust to parameter variations and naturally recovers the position of volumetric structures. In a comparison study with the CPD algorithm it was demonstrated that biomechanically based regularization is key in order to obtain accurate registration results based on sparse sensor data. Furthermore, it was shown that non-linear elasticity models can clearly improve the registration accuracy.
The PBSM approach allows formulating the matching problem as a unified physics-based variational problem. The key advantages of the PBSM method directly result from this formulation: An efficient near real-time numerical solution scheme (even for non-linear elastic models), the matching of partial surfaces as well as the combination with landmark based approaches.
The implementation of the method on multi-core hardware is an important step in order to make it fully real-time capable. This can be done by integrating existing algorithms such as GPU based collision detection [TMY+11] and the previously presented GPU based linear solvers into the framework.
While being a viable registration algorithm in its own right, we especially regard the approach as a powerful component in a larger registration scheme. It has already been shown how any landmark based approach (e.g. texture based tracking) can be naturally embedded into the PBSM algorithm by connecting the known landmarks with stiff springs. In

addition, further research should aim at improving these results by using PBMS in an optimization scheme to estimate the unknown boundary conditions for the biomechanical model at the hidden surfaces (similar to Alterovitz et al. [AGP+06] and Rucker et al. [RWC+13]).

Any intelligent fool can make things bigger, more complex, and more violent. It takes a touch of genius - and a lot of courage - to move in the opposite direction.
— E.F. Schumacher

8. Simulation of surgical cuts

In this section we present a set of numerical methods to model discontinuities in the solution of the elasticity problem without changing the initial grid topology. In the context of real-time intraoperative registration these methods allow adapting the biomechanical model during the operation in the presence of cutting or resection. We start by introducing the eXtended finite element method (X-FEM) and detail an implementation of the approach for corotated finite elements on tetrahedral grids. Subsequently, a formulation is presented that allows modeling arbitrary cuts through tetrahedral elements. For this purpose, the affected elements are enriched with harmonic basis functions that have global support. These functions cause discontinuities at the element boundaries which decrease the accuracy in the standard formulation. In order to overcome this problem we present a novel formulation based on the discontinuous Galerkin (DG) method to embed the enriched elements. A 2D prototype implementation of the technique shows its superior convergence properties in comparison with the standard formulation. Finally, we outline the potential of the aforementioned methods for embedding complex geometries into regular, non-boundary conforming grids. For more information on the basic formulation of the X-FEM formulation for corotated elasticity and the simulation on arbitrary cuts through soft tissue please also refer to the corresponding preprint publications [SSDH13] [PSS+14].

8.1. Modeling discontinuities with the eXtended FE method

8.1.1. The cutting problem for linear elasticity

We extend the formalization of the linear elasticity problem eq. (4.103) to problems that involve a discontinuity (cut). More specifically, we consider the body $\mathcal{B}$ that occupies the region Ω_0 (Fig. 8.1). We again prescribe displacement boundary conditions on Γ_d and force boundary conditions on Γ_n. Additionally, we introduce a cut boundary Γ_c with zero Neumann (force) boundary conditions. Along the lines of the original elasticity problem we require that the different boundaries do not overlap ($\Gamma_D \cap \Gamma_N \cap \Gamma_C = \emptyset$) and that boundary conditions are defined for the whole boundary ($\partial\Omega = \Gamma_D \cup \Gamma_N \cup \Gamma_C$). By defining the function space

$$V_C(\Gamma_C,0) = \{\mathbf{x}|\sigma\mathbf{n} = 0 \qquad \forall \mathbf{x} \in \Gamma_C\} \tag{8.1}$$

in addition to $V_D(\Gamma_D,\overline{\mathbf{u}})$ (eq. 4.100) and $V_N(\Gamma_N,\overline{\mathbf{t}})$ (eq. 4.101) we can formulate the cutting problem for linear elasticity: Find $\mathbf{u} \in C^2(\Omega) \cap C^1(\overline{\Omega}) \cap V_D(\Gamma_D,\overline{\mathbf{u}}) \cap V_N(\Gamma_N,\overline{\mathbf{t}}) \cap V_C(\Gamma_C,0)$ s.t.

$$\mathrm{Div}\sigma + \rho_0\mathbf{g} = \rho_0\ddot{\mathbf{u}} \qquad \forall \mathbf{u} \in \Omega_0 \tag{8.2}$$

$$\epsilon = \frac{1}{2}(\mathrm{Grad}\mathbf{u} + (\mathrm{Grad}\mathbf{u})^T). \tag{8.3}$$

8.1.2. X-FEM based discretization

In agreement with standard FE procedures, we assume that $\mathcal{B}$ is discretized with a tetrahedral mesh (Fig. 8.1 illustrates a 2D example). In order to facilitate an efficient, straight-forward implementation of the extended finite element method (X-FEM), we also approximate the cut through a first order polygonal plane within each element. Furthermore, we lengthen or shorten the cut in such a way that it ends on an element edge. We will see in section 8.2 how to alleviate these restrictions in order to achieve an X-FEM based formulation for arbitrarily shaped cuts.

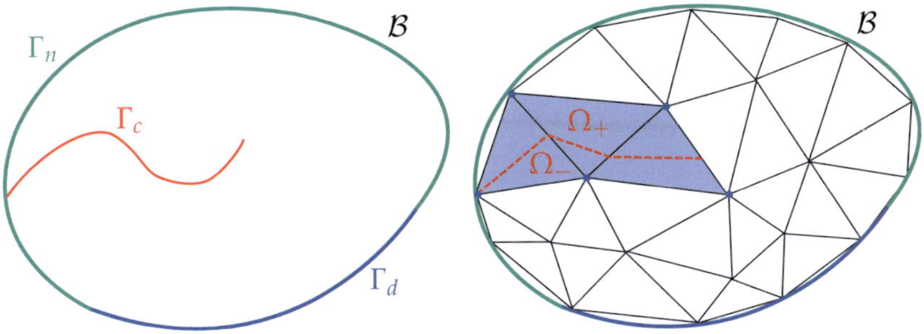

Figure 8.1.: Illustration of the cutting problem in 2D. A body $\mathcal{B}$ with Dirichlet boundary Γ_D and Neumann boundary Γ_N is cut along the stress-free boundary Γ_C (left). This cut is subequently discretized using linear polynomials and the elements that are affected by the cut (blue) are enriched with discontinuous basis functions (right).

The main idea of the X-FEM is to model the discontinuity in the mesh not by changing the mesh topology, but by enriching the basis functions of the finite element space. Thus, the new discontinuous basis functions $\Psi_J = \Psi_J(\mathbf{x})$ are introduced in order to interpolate the displacement

$$\mathbf{u}_h = \sum_{J \in \mathcal{N}_1} \mathcal{U}_J N_J + \sum_{J \in \mathcal{N}_2} \mathcal{A}_J N_J^* \Psi_J \tag{8.4}$$

of the body $\mathcal{B}$. Here, $\mathcal{A}_J \in \mathbb{R}^3$ are additional degrees of freedom that control the size of the gap that is created by the cut. We also introduce the set $\mathcal{N}_1$ of all nodes and the set $\mathcal{N}_2$ that includes all nodes which belong to enriched elements. N_J^* are shape functions that satisfy the previously discussed *partion of unity* condition and the δ-property. Although it is theoretically possible to choose N_J^* that differ from the standard shape functions N_J (e.g. by choosing quadratic N_J^*), we choose $N_J^* = N_J$ in accordance with previous work in the literature. In order to properly define the discontinuous function Ψ_J, the cut is typically represented by a so called level-set function. This allows to define a region above the cut (Ω_+) a region below the cut (Ω_+). In this scenario the *Heaviside* function

$$\Psi_J = H(\mathbf{x}) = \begin{cases} 1, & \mathbf{x} \in \Omega_+ \\ -1, & \mathbf{x} \in \Omega_- \end{cases} \tag{8.5}$$

is an obvious choice for the enrichment function Ψ_J. In order to achieve a more efficient implementation, the interpolation is typically defined in terms of the shifted *Heaviside* function

$$\Psi_J = \frac{H(\mathbf{x}) - H_J(\mathbf{x})}{2}. \tag{8.6}$$

In this formulation, $H_J(\mathbf{x})$ denotes the value of $H(\mathbf{x})$ at the J-th node. When using shifted *Heaviside* functions, the enrichment term is zero at all element nodes. Consequently, the support of the extended part of the interpolation is limited to the enriched element which simplifies the numerical integration during matrix assembly.
In order to use the standard FE discretization scheme, it is convenient to define the extended vector

$$\mathcal{U}^X = [\mathcal{U}_1 \ldots \mathcal{U}_n \, \mathcal{A}_1 \ldots \mathcal{A}_m] \tag{8.7}$$

that contains not only the n nodal displacement vectors, but also the additional $3m$ degrees of freedom $\mathcal{A}_J$. In a similar way, we extend the definition of the basis functions

$$N_J^X = \begin{cases} N_J, & 0 \leq J < n \\ N_J \Psi_J, & n \leq J < n+m \end{cases} \tag{8.8}$$

in order to include the extended interpolation that has been introduced in eq. (8.4). With these definitions, the vector of internal nodal forces

$$\mathbf{f}_I^{int} = \int_{\Omega_0} \sigma_{ik}^X (\nabla N^X)_{kI} \mathrm{dV}_0 \tag{8.9}$$

$$= \int_{\Omega_a} \sigma_{ik}^X (\nabla N^X)_{kI} \mathrm{dV}_0 + \int_{\Omega_b} \sigma_{ik}^X (\nabla N^X)_{kI} \mathrm{dV}_0 \tag{8.10}$$

can be derived in the same way as in the standard FE formulation eq. (5.40). In the above equation, $\Omega_a = \{\mathbf{x}|\Psi(\mathbf{x}) = 1\}$ denotes the region above the cut, while $\Omega_b = \{\mathbf{x}|\Psi(\mathbf{x}) = -1\}$. We also introduce the new variable σ^X for the Cauchy stress tensor in order to explicitly state that

within the support the extended basis functions, the stress is computed using the enriched interpolation eq. (8.4).
It is apparent that the standard FE discretization formalism (e.g. calculation of nodal forces and stiffness matrix) can be directly applied to the extended interpolation eq. (8.4). However, the above equation (8.10) also reveals one important difference that has huge implications on the implementation: Due to the discontinuity inside an element, the numerical integration cannot be performed using Gaussian quadrature (see section 5.2.1). Instead, the two sub-elements that are created below and above the cut have to be integrated independently. If the cut is approximated by a first order polygonal (i.e. straight) plane, there is only a (small) finite number of cases how a tetrahedron can be divided. It is thus possible to divide these sub-elements into tetrahedra based on a case-by-case analysis. Gaussian quadrature can then be performed onto each of these sub-element tetrahedra. Please refer to the preprint publication [SSDH13] for more detailed information on the case-based tetrahedral subdivision scheme.
When inserting the shifted *Heaviside* function into the linear elastic formulation, the elemental stiffness matrices of non-enriched elements remain unchanged. Furthermore, the 24x24 elemental stiffness matrices for the enriched elements are of the form

$$\mathbf{K}^{X,\tau} = \begin{bmatrix} \mathbf{K}^{uu,\tau} & \mathbf{K}^{ua,\tau} \\ \mathbf{K}^{au,\tau} & \mathbf{K}^{aa,\tau} \end{bmatrix}, \tag{8.11}$$

with $\mathbf{K}^{uu,\tau} = \mathbf{K}^{\tau} = K^{\tau}_{ij}$ being the standard 12x12 FE stiffness matrix with the original degrees of freedom. We denote the region that is occupied by element τ with Ω_τ. This allows us to define the volume V of the region Ω_τ as well as the volume V_a of the region $\Omega_+ = \Omega_a \cap \Omega_\tau$ above the cut and the volume V_b of the region $\Omega_- = \Omega_b \cap \Omega_\tau$ below the cut. With this notation the 12x12 sub-matrices of the elemental stiffness matrix is given by

$$
\begin{aligned}
K_{ij}^{uu,\tau} &= K_{ij}^{\tau} \\
K_{ij}^{ua,\tau} &= \left(\frac{V_a}{V}\Psi_{aj} + \frac{V_b}{V}\Psi_{bj}\right) K_{ij}^{\tau} \\
K_{ij}^{au,\tau} &= \left(\frac{V_a}{V}\Psi_{ai} + \frac{V_b}{V}\Psi_{bi}\right) K_{ij}^{\tau} \\
K_{ij}^{au,\tau} &= \left(\frac{V_a}{V}\Psi_{ai}\Psi_{aj} + \frac{V_b}{V}\Psi_{bi}\Psi_{bj}\right) K_{ij}^{\tau}
\end{aligned}
\tag{8.12}
$$

where Ψ_{ai} and Ψ_{bi} denote the value of Ψ_i above and below the cut, respectively.

It is evident from eq. 8.12 that for linear elasticity problems the additional effort for the enriched formulation is primarily reduced to determining the volumes V_a and V_b. As this has to be performed only once when the cut is executed, the overhead of the X-FEM is small in comparison to standard FE. For dynamic problems, the X-FEM mass matrix can be derived in the same way as the stiffness matrix.

If re-meshing techniques are used to model surgical cuts, the creation of small, ill shaped (so called *sliver*) elements can severely reduce the performance and stability of the simulation. In contrast, the X-FEM approach does not suffer from this problem. Even if these kinds of elements are created during the sub-element division process for numerical integration purposes, they do not have an effect on the simulation. However, it is apparent from eq. (8.12) that the stiffness matrix can become ill-conditioned if either V_a or V_b become infinitesimal small. In these cases, the cut runs close to a node. A straight forward solution to this problem is to simply do not enrich the effected node. This approach was first proposed by Sukumar et al. for an X-FEM formulation in two dimensions [SB00]. Experiments with our 3D implementation confirmed that the method introduces only a negligible error while guaranteeing a well-conditioned stiffness matrix. A typical threshold for disabling the enrichment is $\min(V_a, V_b)/V < \epsilon$ with $\epsilon = 10^{-4}$.

8.1.3. X-FEM for corotated elasticity

As discussed in the previous chapters, the linear elasticity model is not suitable in the presence of large deformations. In contrast, corotated elasticity provides a rotation invariant formulation for elastic materials and is a well suited regularization measure for intraoperative registration algorithms. We thus seek to derive an X-FEM formulation for corotated elasticity.
The derivation of the nodal forces and the stiffness matrix for standard corotated elements has already been presented in chapter 5 (see eq. 5.65 and eq. 5.66). If the extended formulation for the degrees of freedom (eq. 8.7) and the basis functions (eq. 8.8) is inserted into this derivative, it is obvious that the elemental nodal forces and the elemental stiffness matrix do not change for non-enriched elements (along the lines of the linear X-FEM discretization). However, the numerical integration becomes much more difficult for the enriched elements. For an accurate corotated formulation, the rotation matrix has to be extracted at every integration point. This introduces a large computational overhead, even if an efficient scheme such as the presented element subdivision technique is used for numerical integration. It should in particular be pointed out that this rotation extraction and the subsequent integration of nodal force and the stiffness matrix assembly has to be carried out for every time step.
In order to significantly reduce this overhead while still maintaining a high accuracy formulation, we rely on the same idea that was presented earlier for the integration of the quadratic tetrahedron: We simply assume the rotation to be constant over a certain region in order to reduce the number of necessary integration points. In the context of the X-FEM the obvious choice is to extract a rotation matrix for each region above and below the cut (see Fig. 8.2).
Starting from eq. (5.65), the extended nodal forces

$$\mathbf{f}_I^{int} = \int_{\Omega_0} R_{im}\sigma_{mk}^{X,CR}(\nabla N^X)_{kI}\mathrm{dV}_0 \tag{8.13}$$

$$= R_{im}^a \int_{\Omega_a} \sigma_{mk}^{X,CR}(\nabla N^X)_{kI}\mathrm{dV}_0 + R_{im}^a \int_{\Omega_b} \sigma_{mk}^{X,CR}(\nabla N^X)_{kI}\mathrm{dV}_0 \tag{8.14}$$

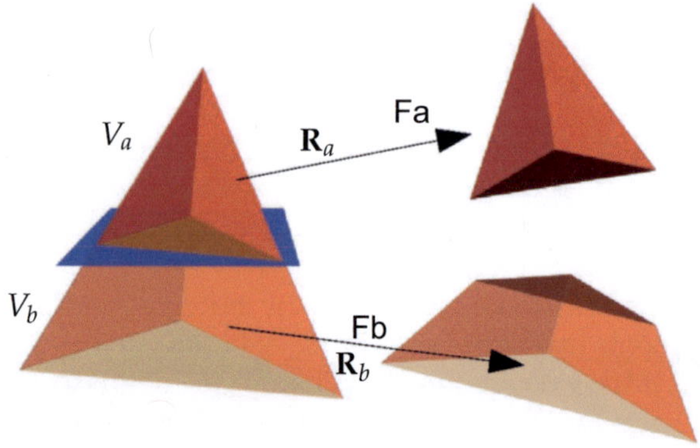

Figure 8.2.: In order to reduce the computational overhead, we only extract one rotation matrix for each region above and below the cut instead of one rotation matrix per integration point [SSDH13].

for the enriched elements are subsequently derived by performing two numerical integration. The elemental stiffness matrix

$$\mathbf{K}^{X,\tau,CR} = \int_{\tau} \mathbf{R} \frac{\partial \hat{\mathbf{f}}_I^{X,int}}{\partial \mathcal{X}_J} \mathbf{R}^T \mathrm{dV}_0 \tag{8.15}$$

$$= \int_{\Omega_a} \mathbf{R}_a \frac{\partial \hat{\mathbf{f}}_I^{X,int}}{\partial \mathcal{X}_J^X} \mathbf{R}_a^T \mathrm{dV}_0 + \int_{\Omega_b} \mathbf{R}_b \frac{\partial \hat{\mathbf{f}}_I^{X,int}}{\partial \mathcal{X}_J^X} \mathbf{R}_b^T \mathrm{dV}_0 \tag{8.16}$$

is computed in the same way. The external load vector as well as the mass matrix in a dynamic problem are the same for linear elasticity and corotated elasticity.

8.1.4. Accuracy validation

The presented X-FEM based approach for surgical cutting was implemented for unstructured tetrahedral grids in a Matlab environment. As explained in the previous sections, a case-by-case subdivision scheme is used for efficient numerical integration. The Newmark time integration scheme is used in a dynamical formulation and the boundary conditions are imposed using the projection based technique presented in chapter 5.

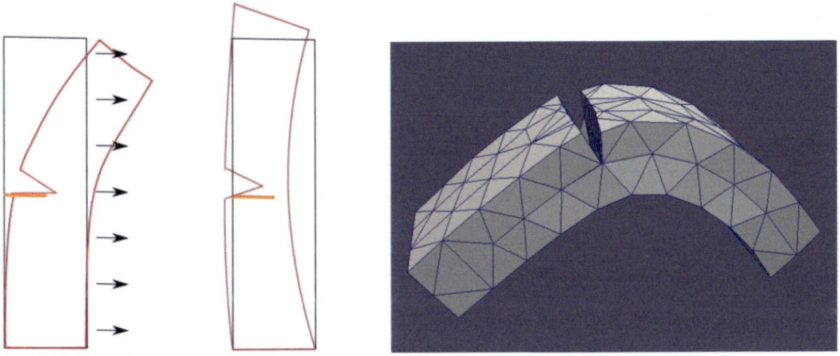

Figure 8.3.: 2D sketch of beam model under gravity load (left) and with displacement boundary conditions that impose a stretching deformation (middle). The 3D model of a beam with a cut under gravity load is shown on the right [SSDH13].

In order to assess the convergence properties of the method, a beam model (dimensions 0.03m$\times$0.06m$\times$0.2m, elastic modulus $E = 300$kPa, Poisson's ration $\nu = 0.35$) with two different deformation patterns is considered (Fig. 8.3). First, we simulate a beam that was cut in the middle under gravity load. Furthermore, we impose a stretching deformation on this model by applying displacement boundary conditions on both ends. A *ground truth* solution for both scenarios is computed using a high resolution grid that perfectly aligns with the cut. Our previously presented SOFA-based implementation of the corotated finite element method is used to compute this reference solution. In contrast, the mesh for the corotated X-FEM is chosen in such a way that the cut always runs through different elements. For the sake of the convergence analysis, we use a structured tetrahedral grid and sequentially double the resolution for each spatial direction.
The convergence analysis (Fig. 8.4) shows that for the first scenario, the X-FEM based approach achieves a higher accuracy than the standard FEM on a perfectly aligned grid. In contrast, it does not perform as well for the other deformation pattern. However, the convergence behavior is

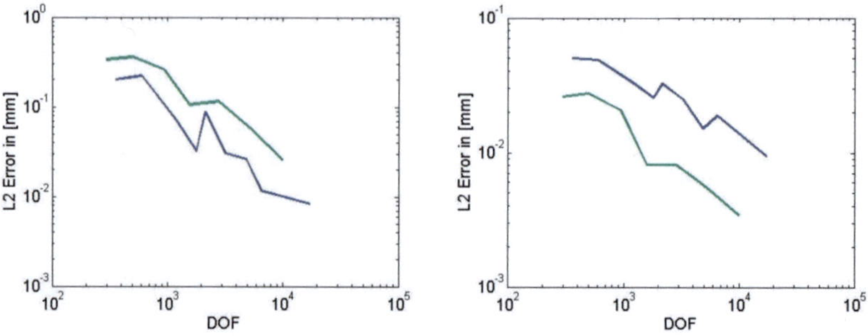

Figure 8.4.: Results of the convergence analysis for beam under gravity (left) and the stretched beam (right). The error of the X-FEM implementation is shown in blue, while the standard FEM solution is marked blue [SSDH13].

very similar to the standard FE approach. This is a very promising result as the X-FEM is competitive to a standard FE on a grid that is perfectly aligned to the cut (perfect re-meshing). For more complex cuts that are meshed on-the-fly, the performance of standard FE usually degrade significantly.

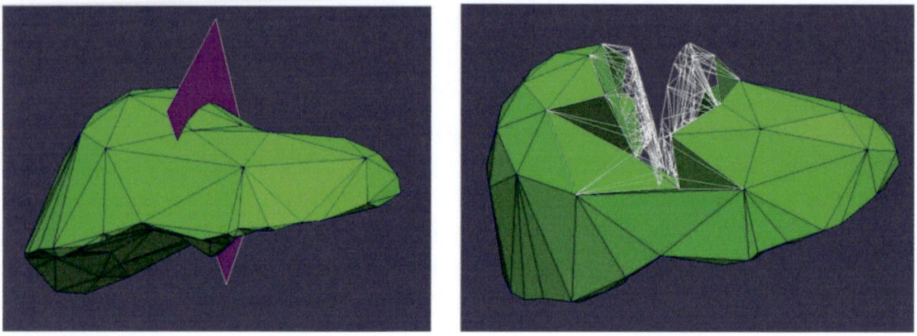

Figure 8.5.: Cutting of a liver model using corotated X-FEM [SSDH13].

The developed cutting method was also applied to more complex geometries (Fig. 8.5). It is important to point out that in order to achieve a good visualization, it is necessary to split the elements that are affected by the cut. In this context, we use the same elemental subdivision that was

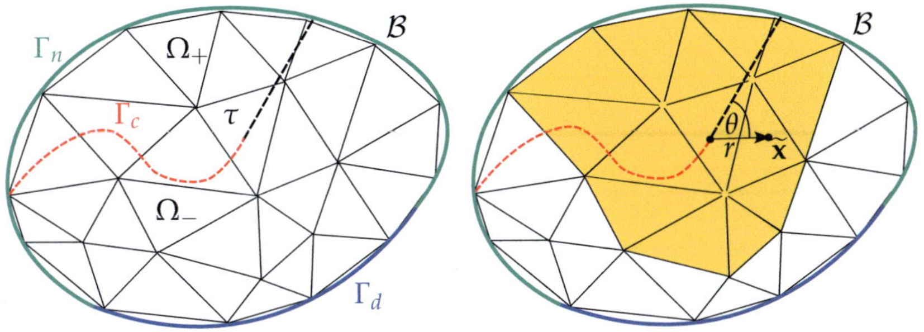

Figure 8.6.: A stress-free cut through the body $\mathcal{B}$ with Dirichlet boundary Γ_D and Neumann boundary Γ_N ends in element τ (left). In order to model the wedge-shaped opening of the cut, a 2D polar coordinate system is introduced in order to define additional harmonic basis functions (right).

constructed for the numerical integration scheme for the visualization of the cut.

8.2. Simulating arbitrary cuts in soft tissue

It was shown in the previous section how an enrichment of the finite element interpolation with the shifted Heaviside function can be used in order to model cuts that run completely through an element. This type of enrichment is usually referred to as sign enrichment. We also detailed the arising X-FEM formulation and showed how it can be implemented on tetrahedral grids, if the cut is approximated by a first order polygonal (i.e. straight) plane. In the following section we will show how arbitrary cuts can be modeled. For this purpose we first introduce another type of enrichment that allows to model cuts that end within an element. Furthermore, a simple numerical integration technique is introduced that allows to derive the nodal forces and elemental stiffness matrices for arbitrarily shaped cuts.

8.2.1. Branch enrichment

We consider an arbitrarily shaped cut through the body $\mathcal{B}$ (Fig. 8.6) that ends within the element τ (Fig. 8.6). In a 3D setting, the end of the cut is a line that runs through τ. This line is also called the cutfront CF^{τ}. In the 2D example depicted in Fig. 8.6 the cutfront is reduced to a point. The cutfront has a direction, which is given by the tangent to the cut. The cutfront can be progressed along this direction in order to virtually extend the cut through the whole body $\mathcal{B}$ (dashed black line in Fig. 8.6).
The termination of the cut within the element τ and the resulting wedge-shaped opening of the cut cannot be modeled using the previously presented sign enrichment approach. Instead, additional enrichment functions have to be used. It is intuitively clear, that these enrichment functions will have rotational symmetries along the direction of the cutfront (dashed black line in Fig. 8.6). As these functions can be constant along the cutfront, Moës et al. proposed to use the 2D polar coordinate system (r,θ) to express the values of the function [MDB99]. Here, r is the distance of an arbitrary point $\widetilde{\mathbf{x}}$ to the cutfront and the θ denotes the angle between the distance vector and the direction of the cutfront (see Fig. 8.6). Moës proposed to use the four so called asymptotic crack tip functions (ACTF)

$$F_1(r,\theta) = \sqrt{r}\sin(\theta/2) \tag{8.17}$$

$$F_2(r,\theta) = \sqrt{r}\cos(\theta/2) \tag{8.18}$$

$$F_3(r,\theta) = \sqrt{r}\sin(\theta/2)\sin(\theta) \tag{8.19}$$

$$F_4(r,\theta) = \sqrt{r}\cos(\theta/2)\sin(\theta) \tag{8.20}$$

as additional basis functions for elements that are partially cut. This allows us to formulate the new extended FE interpolation

$$\mathbf{u}_h = \sum_{J\in\mathcal{N}_1} \mathcal{U}_J N_J + \sum_{J\in\mathcal{N}_2} \mathcal{A}_J N_J \Psi_J + \sum_{J\in\mathcal{N}_3} N_J \sum_{L=1}^{4} \mathcal{C}_{JL} F_L(r,\theta) \tag{8.21}$$

for fully enriched elements. The enrichment of the interpolation with ACTFs is also called branch enrichment. The additional degrees of freedom are denoted with $\mathcal{C}_{JL}$ and the set $\mathcal{N}_3$ denotes all nodes that are branch enriched.

We point out that the support of the ACTFs is not limited to the enriched elements, but also includes the neighboring elements. Furthermore the branch enrichment term violates the partition of unity eq. (5.28) and the δ-property eq. (5.27). Consequently, the convergence rate of the X-FEM is decreased, if only the direct neighbors of the partially cut element are enriched with the ACTFs. In order to reduce these so called parasitic effects, a larger neighborhood of nodes around τ can be enriched (i.e. added to $\mathcal{N}_3$). However, this introduces 4 additional DOF for each branch enriched node and thus considerably increases the computational overhead. We also note that these nodes in a completely cut element which are shared with a partially cut element (and are thus already branch enriched), are not additionally enriched with a Heaviside basis function.
For a typical 3D simulation, the cut is given by a triangulated surface. In this context, the geometric computation of the cutfront for each element using appropriate collision detection schemes is challenging. This is also true for the computation of the local coordinate system that properly defines the ACTFs. For an in-depth explanation of these important implementation details please refer to the corresponding preprint publication[PSS$^+$14]-

8.2.2. Accurate numerical integration

In order to derive the nodal force vector and the elemental stiffness matrices, we follow the approach that was outlined in the previous section: First, the vector of all DOFs and the vector of all basis functions is extended. Then, these extensions are inserted in the discretization formalism that is already known from the standard finite element technique. As this procedure is completely analogous to the previously presented derivation, we do not outline the details here. However, it is important to note that the numerical integration has to be handled differently in the presence of ACTF.
As the ACTFs are no polynomial functions, they cannot be exactly integrated using Gaussian quadrature, even when the presented element subdivision scheme is used. We use a straight forward integration scheme to overcome this problem: We simply embed a higher resolution structured grid into each enriched elements and sample the displacement function at the nodes of the structured grid. Furthermore, the polar coor-

dinates (r,θ) are evaluated at each sample point in order to compute the value of the ACTFs for each integration point. The big drawback of the method is that many integration points have to be used, thus rendering it very computationally intensive. However, for the corotated X-FEM we again only distinguish between a rotation above and below the crack. This means that the complex integration procedure has to be performed only once; if the course of the cut is known beforehand, it can even be done in a pre-computing step. For each time step, only the two regions above and below the cut have to be rotated accordingly and assembled into the stiffness matrix. This oversampling method can also be used for all sign enriched elements. In this case, it is not necessary to assume that the cut is given as a piecewise linear plane. Instead, arbitrarily shaped cuts can be simulated. The resolution of these cuts is controlled by the resolution of the oversampling grid.

8.2.3. Accuracy validation

The described X-FEM for the simulation of arbitrary cuts in elastic models was implemented in the SOFA framework. In order to assess the convergence properties of the method we again consider the two model problems described in the previous section (Fig. 8.3). In this scenario, we limit the analysis to linear elastic models. This allows us to compute the ground truth solution with the commercial Abaqus finite element method on a structured tetrahedral mesh that is perfectly aligned with the cut. We use an unstructured tetrahedral grid for the X-FEM based computations (see Fig. 8.7). This implies that there are elements that have to be partially cut.

The convergence analysis (Fig. 8.8) shows that the X-FEM based approach is considerably more accurate for the same number of DOF than the standard FE technique. This difference can be partly attributed to the fact that an unstructured grid can be used for the X-FEM computations. This usually does not suffer as much from volume locking as structured tetrahedral grids. Furthermore, the results indicate that although the X-FEM method is more accurate for the analyzed resolutions, the convergence rate of the standard FE technique might be higher. However, it is still reasonable to conclude that an X-FEM technique based on sign enrichment and branch enrichment cannot only model arbitrarily shaped

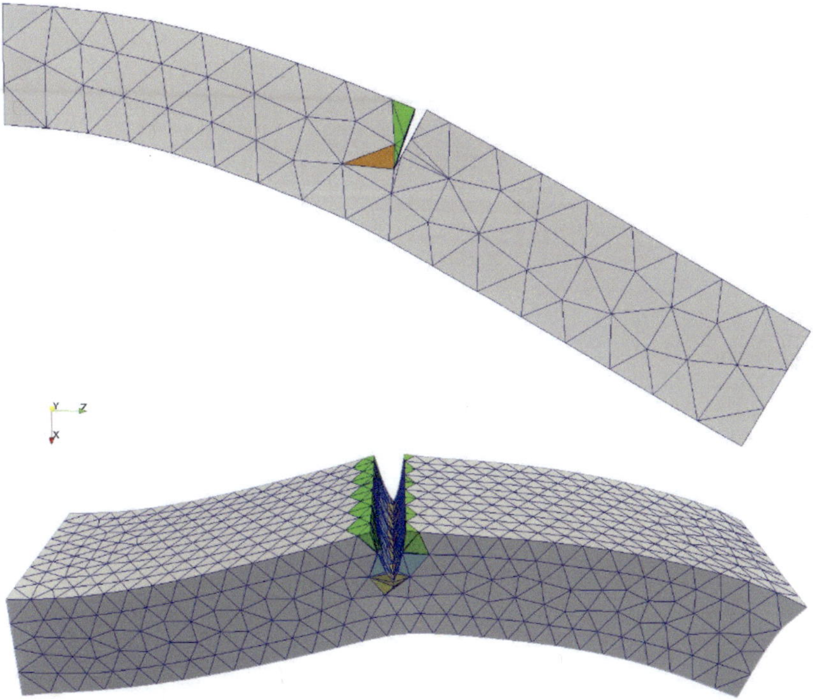

Figure 8.7.: Cutting simulation of a beam under gravity load (top) and stretched beam (bottom) using the X-FEM technique [PSS+14].

cuts, but also performs at least as good as a well meshed standard FE approach in terms of accuracy per number of DOFs.
An example of an arbitrarily shaped cut through a more complex geometry can be seen in Fig. 8.9. Here, a liver is divided by a wave shaped cut.

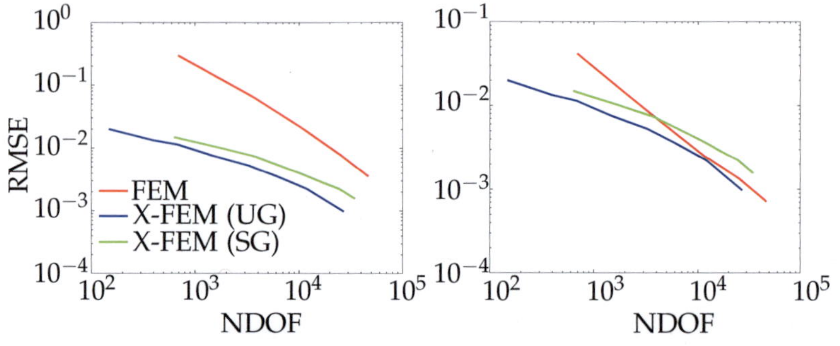

Figure 8.8.: Results of the convergence analysis for beam under gravity (left) and the stretched beam (right). The X-FEM based technique consistently outperforms the standard FE approach for the analyzed meshes [PSS+14].

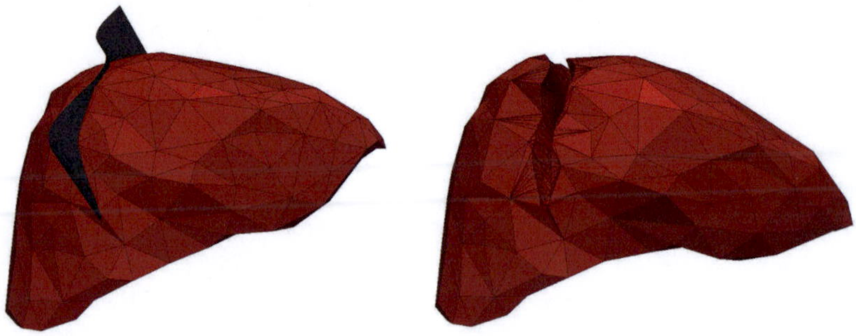

Figure 8.9.: Arbitrarily shaped cut through a liver model using X-FEM with sign and branch enrichment.

8.3. Efficient embedding of enriched elements

It has already been discussed that the branch enrichment violates the partition of unity. This leads to a decrease in accuracy. One way to overcome this problem is to enrich further elements near the crack tip. However, this approach introduces a lot more degrees of freedom and is thus unsuitable in the real-time setting. A more elegant way to remedy this problem is to embed the branch enriched elements into the standard

finite element grid using the discontinuous Galerkin (DG) method. This finite element method allows the shape functions to be discontinuous at the element boundaries.
In this section preliminary work towards a hybrid DG-FEM / X-FEM method is presented. We outline the main ideas of the DG method, show how it can be applied to problems in linear elasticity and present qualitative results from a prototype implementation for 2D problems. For a more detailed introduction to the DG method we refer to the introductory text by Cockburn [BC99] or the corresponding diploma thesis publications by Pfau [PSDH10] and Huber [Hub11]. The presented DG formulation for linear elasticity is based on the work of Lew et al. [TEL06] [LNSO04].

8.3.1. The Discontinuous Galerkin method

In contrast to the classic conformal Galerkin (CG) method, the discontinuous Galerkin (DG) approach allows discontinuities in the solution at the element boundaries. This has important consequences for the problem formulation and the finite element discretization. First of all, the space V_h of all DG solutions is not a subspace of the space V of all continuous solutions. This means that statements about the uniqueness and the existence of solutions do not carry over from the continuous to the discrete formulation. Furthermore, the weak formulation of the elasticity problem cannot be derived from Cauchy's equation of motion in the way that was demonstrated in section 5.1.1. In particular, it is not possible to apply the divergence theorem to the whole region Ω_0 as shown in (eq. 5.4). In contrast, it has to be applied to each element independently and surface integrals remain in the formulation that have to be integrated into the stiffness matrix. These surface integrals can be regarded as interaction forces that couple the different elements whereas in CG-FEM the coupling is achieved through the continuity condition.
In the upcoming sections we present a DG formulation that builds on the definition of a so called discontinuous Galerkin derivative D_{DG}. Based on this definition, we can define a variational formulation for the elasticity problem that can be discretized using the well-known standard FE procedure. In order to facilitate a clean description of the method, some terminology has to be introduced.

For all elements τ, the set of all element faces $\Gamma = \bigcup_{\tau \in \mathcal{M}} \partial\tau$ is divided into the set

$$\Gamma_I = e \in \Gamma \setminus \partial\Omega_0 \tag{8.22}$$

of all inner faces as well as the set of all element faces Γ_d on the Dirichlet boundary and the set of all faces Γ_n on the Neumann boundary. Here, e denotes the face that is shared by elements τ_+ and τ_-. The associated face normal $\mathbf{n}$ is oriented outwards of τ_-.
V_h^τ denotes a discrete vector space of smooth scalar functions in the element τ (e.g. the set of linear polynomials in a tetrahedral element). With this definition, the DG finite element space can be expressed through $V_h = \prod_{\tau \in \mathcal{M}} V_h^\tau$. The extension of the scalar function space V_h to the space of d-dimensional vector valued functions is called V_h^d and will later be used to approximate the displacement field. In the same way, we define the function space W_h^d to approximate a gradient to a function in V_h. Later, we will also use the tensor-valued function space $W_h^{d \times d}$ to approximate the deformation gradient.
It is clear that the functions in V_h are double-valued on the inner faces Γ_I. In order to a facilitate a mapping scheme to a singular value, we define the jump $[\![\cdot]\!]$ and the average operator $\{\cdot\}$ for the functions $v \in V_h$ and $\mathbf{z} \in W_h^d$:

$$[\![v]\!] = v^- - v^+ \qquad \text{and} \qquad \{v\} = \frac{1}{2}(v^- + v^+) \tag{8.23}$$

$$[\![\mathbf{z}]\!] = \mathbf{z}^- - \mathbf{z}^+ \qquad \text{and} \qquad \{\mathbf{z}\} = \frac{1}{2}(\mathbf{z}^- + \mathbf{z}^+) \tag{8.24}$$

On the boundary faces $e \in \Gamma \setminus \Gamma_I$ we additionally define

$$[\![v]\!] = v \qquad \text{and} \qquad \{\mathbf{z}\} = \mathbf{z}. \tag{8.25}$$

Several possibilities exist to define the singular value $\hat{v}$ of the solution on the element faces. The choice of this so called numerical flux determines how the elements are coupled together. In this work we choose the flux $\hat{v}(v) = \hat{v}_0(v) + \hat{v}_\partial(v)$ with

$$\hat{v}_0(v) = \begin{cases} \{v\} & \text{on } \Gamma_I \\ 0 & \text{on } \Gamma_d \\ 0 & \text{on } \Gamma_n \end{cases}, \qquad \hat{v}_\partial(v) = \begin{cases} 0 & \text{on } \Gamma_I \\ \overline{v} & \text{on } \Gamma_d \\ v & \text{on } \Gamma_n \end{cases} \tag{8.26}$$

that was proposed by Bassi and Rebay [BR97]. This flux formulation allows to impose the Dirichlet boundary values $\overline{v}$ in a weak way.

8.3.2. Weak Discontinuous Galerkin derivative

As mentioned before, it is possible to enforce the inter-element coupling through surface forces. However, this method requires the computation of additional surface integrals during the stiffness matrix assembly. A more efficient way is to define so called lifting operators that map the surface integrals to a volume integral. Following the work of Arnold et al. the lifting operator $\mathbf{O}$[1] can be derived by inserting a DG discretization into the Poisson equation [ABCM02]. $\mathbf{O}$ is then defined by the equation

$$\int_{\Omega_0} \mathbf{O}(v) \cdot \mathbf{z} = -\int_{\Gamma} v \otimes \mathbf{n} \cdot \{\mathbf{z}\}, \tag{8.27}$$

where $\otimes$ denotes the tensor product in case v is vector valued ($v \in V_h^d$). It is important to note that $\mathbf{O} : L^2(\Gamma) \mapsto W_h^d$ is a linear operator with small, compact support. For implementation purposes it is efficient to break down $\mathbf{O}$ to elemental contributions and accordingly define the elemental lifting operator $\mathbf{O}^\tau$ through the equation

$$\int_{\tau} \mathbf{O}^\tau(v) \cdot \mathbf{z} = -\int_{\partial\tau} v \otimes \mathbf{n} \cdot \{\mathbf{z}\}. \tag{8.28}$$

By inserting the finite element approximation for v and $\mathbf{z}$ in the above equation, the matrix representation for $\mathbf{O}^\tau$ can be derived (see [Hub11] for details). If standard nodal shape functions are used, the support (and thus the size of the matrix representation) includes all nodes of τ and the nodes that share a face with τ (e.g. a total of 16 nodes in a linear tetrahedral grid).
The lifting operator allows defining the DG derivative operator

$$D_{DG} v = \nabla v + \mathbf{O}([\![v]\!]) - \mathbf{O}([\![\hat{v}_\partial(v)]\!]) \tag{8.29}$$

which approximates ∇v. Here, the operator is defined on the scalar function v and consequently we have $D_{DG} : V_h \mapsto W_h^d$. However, the extension

[1] usually denoted $\mathbf{R}$ in the literature, we use $\mathbf{O}$ to avoid confusion with the rotation matrix

to vector valued functions is straight forward: For the displacement field $\mathbf{u}_h \in V_h^d$ we define $D_{DG}\mathbf{u}_h = \mathbf{e}_i \otimes (D_{DG}u_j)$, where $\mathbf{e}_i$ denotes the unit vectors in $\mathbb{R}^d$. In this context the lifting operator $\mathbf{O}(\mathbf{u}_h) = \mathbf{e}_i \otimes \mathbf{O}(u_j)$ is extended in the same way and we obtain $\mathbf{O} : [L^2(\Gamma)]^d \mapsto W_h^{d\times d}$.

8.3.3. DG-FEM for linear elasticity

The definition of the DG derivative opens up a very elegant way to derive the DG-FEM discretization for elastic materials. We simply insert the DG derivative operator D_{DG} instead of the standard gradient operator ∇ into the variational form eq. (5.15). For linear elastic materials, the infinitesimal strain tensor eq. (4.21) thus becomes

$$\epsilon^{DG} = \frac{1}{2}(D_{DG}\mathbf{u}_h + (D_{DG}\mathbf{u}_h)^T) \tag{8.30}$$

and the corresponding Cauchy stress tensor σ^{DG} can be computed by inserting the strain tensor into the material law. This readily yields the variation of the internal elastic energy

$$D_{\delta\mathbf{u}_h}\Pi(\mathbf{u}_h)_{int} = \int_{\Omega_0} \sigma^{DG} : \delta\epsilon^{DG} \mathrm{dV}_0. \tag{8.31}$$

However, due to the non-conformity of the discretization the ensuing variational problem can have multiple solutions, which often causes instabilities in the simulation. In order to overcome this problem, a stabilization term has to be added to the formulation. The basic idea is to add an energy term that punishes the discontinuities (*jumps*) at the element boundaries to the total energy of the system. A straight forward approach is to simply integrate the squared *jumps* over the elements' faces. The stabilization energy

$$\Pi(\mathbf{u}_h)_{stab} = \frac{\tilde{\beta}}{h}\int_{\Gamma} [\![\mathbf{u}_h - \hat{v}(\mathbf{u}_h)]\!] \cdot [\![\mathbf{u}_h - \hat{v}(\mathbf{u}_h)]\!] \cdot \mathrm{dS} \tag{8.32}$$

is obtained by scaling this term with a constant $\tilde{\beta}$ and the characteristic element length h. If the constant $\tilde{\beta}$ is chosen to be very high, the DG-FEM gives nearly identical results to the CG-FEM. In practice, the choice of $\tilde{\beta}$

heavily depends on the material parameters and can be quite difficult for the stabilization term introduced above. That is why we use an extended stabilization term proposed by Lew et al. that also scales the energy with the material parameters [LNSO04] in our implementation.
The discrete matrix formulation of the DG-FEM can be derived with the same formalism that has already been presented for the CG-FEM, for details we again refer to [Hub11].

8.3.4. Embedding of enriched elements using DG-FEM

In order to motivate an efficient DG-FEM formulation for the embedding of *branch* enriched elements, we briefly discuss the most important differences between DG-FEM and CG-FEM. First of all, each DG-FEM element has its own degrees of freedom, whereas nodes (i.e. DOF) are shared between the elements in a standard FE discretization. For unstructured tetrahedral grids a DG-FEM discretization can thus easily have an order of magnitude more DOF than the CG-FEM variant. Furthermore, the elemental stiffness matrices are much bigger due to the larger support of the lifting operator in comparison with standard nodal shape functions. Consequently, the global stiffness matrix has higher connectivity. Due to these two properties, the DG-FEM is typically not as computationally efficient as the CG-FEM [TEL06].
For this reason, we do not use a full DG mesh in our implementation. Instead, we use a DG-FEM formulation only for the enriched elements and their respective neighbors. The coupling of DG and CG elements can be achieved by slightly altering the lifting operator **O**: When computing the matrix representation of **O** according to (eq. 8.28) we simply do not integrate over these element faces that are shared with full CG elements. Consequently, we compute a full lifting operator for each branch enriched element. For each neighbor of these elements, we choose nodal shape functions and limit the support of **O** to the element's DOF as well as the enriched element's DOF.
Due to this approach, the number of additional DOF is negligible (especially in comparison with the added DOF due to the branch enrichment). However, we can still leverage the crucial advantage of the DG discretization where necessary: As the solution does not need to be continuous at the element boundaries, the choice of basis functions is not restricted to standard nodal shape functions. Instead, a wide variety of basis func-

tions can be employed. In our specific application we use this freedom to efficiently embed asymptotic crack tip functions into the discretization.

8.3.5. Accuracy validation

The outlined DG-FEM approach was implemented in Matlab for two dimensional, linear elastic problems. The results show that the proposed lifting operator based scheme to embed DG elements into a CG-FEM dominated mesh is accurate and straight forward to implement. Furthermore, different stabilization terms were analyzed (Fig. 8.10). It was observed that the choice of the stabilization term has a strong effect on the solution: If the stabilization is too low, the simulation becomes unstable. However, if the stabilization is too high, the simulation essentially behaves like CG-FEM based discretization and all advantages of the DG approach are lost. For non-linear elastic problems, finding the optimal stabilization parameter proved to be difficult in our analysis and still is an open area of research [ECL08]. However, for linear elastic problems (and consequently also for corotated elasticity) the material dependent stabilization term proved to be very stable. A stabilization parameter of $\beta = 10$ was a good choice for all analyzed materials and scenarios.

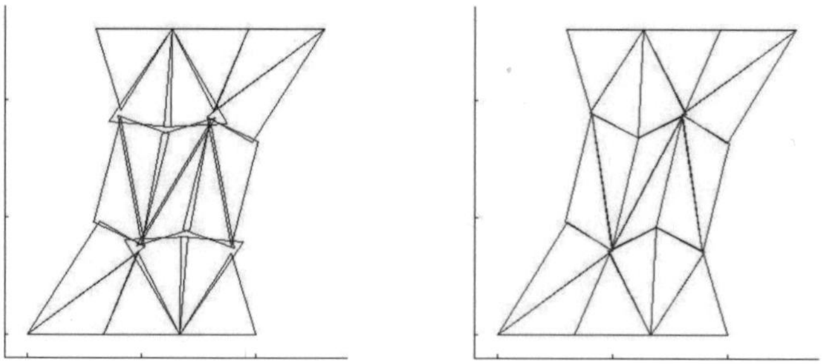

Figure 8.10.: Very low resolution rectangle under displacement boundary conditions and its DG-FEM solution without stabilization term (left) and with a material dependent stabilization term (right) [Hub11].

Two model problems were considered in order to assess the convergence behavior of the proposed hybrid X-FEM/DG-FEM for simulating arbitrary cuts in elastic materials. In particular, the accuracy was assessed for different stabilization parameters. A moderate stabilization leads to a significantly more accurate solution than a very high stabilization parameter (which reproduces the pure CG-FEM solution).

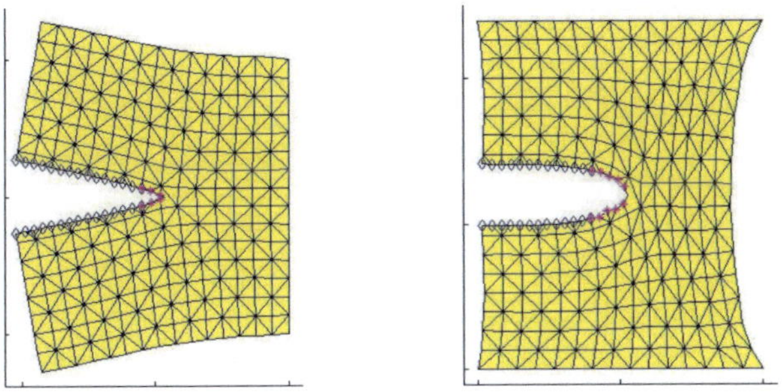

Figure 8.11.: 2D rectangle with cut: With fixed boundary on the right and surface loads on the top and bottom (left) as well as with displacement BCs on the top and bottom (right) [Hub11].

8.4. Towards voxel based simulation

In the previous sections, we have analyzed a set of new methods to simulate cuts in soft tissue. In contrast to classical re-meshing based approaches, these techniques allow to model the cut without changing the underlying grid topology. Computational intensive re-meshing is thus not necessary for real-time cutting and the creation of unstable *sliver* elements are avoided. In addition, the results demonstrate that the X-FEM based approach can be more efficient than the standard FE approach in terms of accuracy per number of degrees of freedom. This is in particular true, if a DG-FEM scheme is used in order to embed the enriched elements.

On a more general level, the presented approach can be interpreted as a paradigm shift in comparison to re-meshing techniques. Whereas classical FE methods seeks to accurately model the problem by using computational grids that closely resemble the geometry, the presented methods operate on meshes that do not need to be fitted to the geometry. Instead, more complex basis functions are used to construct the finite element space. This paradigm also influences the implementation and computational properties of the finite element techniques. In classical FEM, the numerical complexity is primarily given by the number of degrees of freedom. It was demonstrated by our experiments that non-fitted methods can achieve a better efficiency in terms of DOF due to the special basis functions. However, this comes at a price: The numerical integration of the enriched elements is much more complex; not only from an implementation point of view, but also in terms of computational complexity.

Techniques that evolve around the discussed DG-FEM and X-FEM ultimately allow efficiently simulating problems with meshes that do not resemble the actual geometry. This helps to remove the difficult meshing step in the biomechanical simulation workflow. Recently, some groups have demonstrated that similar methods based on the DG-FEM can be used for efficient simulation of elastic problems [RLB09] [BE09]. The idea to shift some complexity into the numerical integration step in order to reduce the number of degrees of freedom bears strong resemblance with the idea of *composite* FEM that has recently become popular in the computer graphics community [NKJF09] [WDW13].

An FE approach based on non-matching boundary grids can be especially beneficial to solve biomechanical problems on massive parallel hardware. First of all, these techniques allow the use of structured, rectangular grids that result in data structures that are well suited for GPU based computations. Furthermore, biomechanical simulations are constructed from voxel-based tomographic images anyway. Thus, the segmented geometry can be readily embedded into a coarser computational grid and the numerical integration could be directly performed on the voxel level.

Life is cheap. It's the accessories that kill you!

— Anonymous

9. Biomechanical modeling workflow and CAS validation

Within the previous chapters a novel approach for biomechanically based real-time intraoperative soft tissue simulation was presented. In order to translate biomechanics based methods into clinical routine and in order to speed up the development of such methods, efficient tools for constructing patient-specific biomechanical models are necessary. Currently, no solution exists that allows combining and accessing the necessary tools such as segmentation and meshing algorithms in an intuitive and easy way. In the upcoming section, we propose a flexible, XML-based concept called the Medical Simulation Markup Language (MSML) in order to overcome this problem.
An efficient and meaningful accuracy validation is another important aspect for the efficient development of clinically viable CAS components. In order to improve this critical development step, we propose a novel approach for manufacturing mechanically accurate soft tissue phantoms. Furthermore, numerics (*in silico*) based validation strategies are discussed and we introduce Open-CAS, a web platform for open data in the context of CAS validation.

9.1. The Medical Simulation Markup Language

Modeling and simulation of human organs by means of continuum mechanics is not only a promising approach for soft tissue registration in the context of computer assisted surgery. The technique has also become an important tool in diagnostics (e.g. for cardiovascular diseases), intervention planning and training. The construction of patient-specific

biomechanical models from tomographic data is a non-trivial workflow that can roughly be divided into six steps. Having segmented relevant anatomical structures from tomographic data, a surface mesh is constructed from these segmented images. Different pre-processing operators (e.g. smoothing, coarsening) are usually applied in order to simplify the subsequent construction of the volumetric grid. Thereafter material properties, boundary conditions and contact surfaces are defined and the simulation is performed. Finally, the data is post-processed for visualization or diagnostic purposes.
Although a diverse ecosystem of software tools exists for each of these steps, there is currently no solution that allows combining and accessing these tools in an intuitive and easy way. In contrast, the available software often even uses incompatible data formats. Whereas this is a negligible problem for surface processing (.stl works well here), numerous different formats exist for volumetric meshes. When it comes to describing material properties, boundary conditions or simulation parameters it even seems as if every tool has its own format.
The complexity of the available tools for the construction of patient-specific biomechanical models is a major barrier for a widespread adoption of these procedures into clinical research. Furthermore, the lack of standards concerning interfaces and data formats makes prototyping medical simulation workflows for specific applications very time consuming.
In order to overcome these problems, we have developed the Medical Simulation Markup Language (MSML). This XML-based scheme allows describing all stages of the simulation workflow. New components (so called operators) can easily be included by providing a simple XML-based description. The MSML acts as a middleware between all tools used in the modeling pipeline and can perform dependency and compatibility checking on the workflow components. Additionally, the MSML allows describing a biomechanical model including all relevant information such as a mesh description as well as the material model and boundary conditions. This unified description can be easily exported to different simulation engines or FE solvers.
In the following sections the XML-based concept for describing the biomechanical workflow is outlined. Furthermore, we present a concrete implementation and show different examples that highlight the flexibility, robustness and ease-of-use of the approach. The presentation is based

on the corresponding publication [SSS+14]. It should be noted that the MSML concept is still in development and updated information can also be found on the MSML website [1].

9.1.1. Flexible XML-based description concepts

Workflow description

Each stage in the simulation workflow is associated with certain data types such as images, segmentation masks, meshes or an indices list. MSML allows to link data types through so-called operators. An operator can be either defined between different stages (e.g. segmentation algorithms link tomographic data to surface meshes, meshing algorithms link surface meshes to volume meshes) or between data that belongs to the same stage (e.g. surface mesh smoother, file format converter). For each operator, an XML-file defines its input and output data types, the data formats, all operator parameters and some information on how the operator can be executed (Fig. 9.1). The data format and data type descriptions must be present in the MSML alphabet. This enables a compatibility checking between operators and their input and output elements. If incompatible data formats are detected, but the same data type is used, the system can use the list of known operators to suggest an appropriate conversion operator. Data types and operators can be added to the alphabet by simply providing an XML-file that describes the corresponding executable or library. In this way it becomes very easy to integrate established software tools into the MSML scheme. MSML thus acts as a middleware between all tools used in the modeling pipeline.

Biomechanical model description

A similar XML-based approach is used to describe the actual biomechanical model. Here, we additionally defined so-called fixed elements; these elements remain the same for all biomechanics simulations regardless if they are FE-based or not, if solid mechanic or fluid dynamic problems are considered. The *physicsModel* contains the *mesh* and several *materialRegions*, which denote material models for different areas that are specified by *indexGroups*. The *physicsElement* might also contain a *contactModel*.

[1] github.com/CognitionGuidedSurgery/msml

The element *simulationSteps* contains the constraints, loads and boundary conditions which can be prescribed for each *step*. In addition to the *physicsModel*, the object also holds a *visualModel* and *postProcessingRequests*. The *MSMLScene* is divided into several *objects* and also contains global parameters about the solver (i.e. ODE or linear systems solver used). All other components of the final MSML alphabet (e.g. material models, mesh types) are defined by a hierarchy of XML files. This results in a remarkable flexibility. New material models (Fig. 9.1), boundary condition types or even completely different physical behavior can be defined by just adding an XML file.

```
<mesherTetgen type="operator" moduleName="TetOp"
methodName="createVolMeshTet" >
 <inputNames> <surfaceMesh/> </inputNames>
 <outputName> <mesh/> </outputName>
 <inputTypes> <triangularMesh/> </inputTypes>
 <outputTypes> <linearTetMesh/> </outputTypes>
 <inputFormats> <file.vtk/> </inputFormats>
 <outputFormats> <file.vtk/> </outputFormats>
 <parameters>
 <preserveBoundary type="bool"/> </parameters>
</mesherTetgen>
```

Figure 9.1.: Definition of a meshing operator in MSML.

The idea behind the unified MSML description is to allow for an easy export to different physics engines or FE solvers. However, each of these export targets might only support a subset of the MSML alphabet. That is why every export operator holds a tree of compatible nodes. This allows for an easy compatibility checking scheme that ensures the consistency between the MSML description and the solver.

9.1.2. Implementation

The MSML scheme was implemented as a hybrid Python/C++ library. All high level functions such as XML-parsing, compatibility checking and operator calls are performed by the Python part. Operators can either be executed as a function call or as a command line tool. This allows for a flexible integration of 3rd party tools. The current operator collection includes different operators based on the visualization toolkit (VTK), CGAL, Gmsh, VCGLib as well as Tetgen. These operators provide functionality such as surface mesh size reduction, linear and quadratic tetrahedral mesh generation, extraction of point and element indices based on different criteria, as well as post processing operations such as mesh coloring and mesh comparison. These operators are implemented in C++ for performance reasons. While it is possible to store all data associated with a MSML model into a single XML-file, it is often more efficient to leave image and mesh data in their native formats and just reference it by filename. All referenced data is copied to a single folder, which can be compressed to reduce storage requirements. In our reference implementation, we use the data types (e.g. for images and meshes) from the visualization toolkit (VTK), but it is of course possible to use different formats thanks to the flexibility of the MSML operators.

9.1.3. Examples workflows and applications

Several different application scenarios were used in order to develop and validate the Medical Simulation Markup Language. In the following paragraphs two of these scenarios are presented. They can be downloaded along with other examples from the MSML website. The Python implementation as well as all specifications and XML schemata are also available for download under an open source license.

Validation of FE algorithms during development

Validation is an important and often time consuming step in FE development. Typically, this means comparing the results obtained using novel implementations and methods with standard techniques. The MSML can not only simplify the generation of suitable testing scenarios, but can also export the same scenario to different FE solvers and allows comparing the results. We used MSML to validate a quadratic co-rotated tetrahedral FE for real-time soft tissue simulation [SRD+11]. A MSML operator chain was used to fully automatically extract a low-resolution quadratic tetrahedral computational mesh from a high-resolution surface mesh of a segmented human liver (Fig. 9.2, 9.3). Furthermore a fully non-linear version of the model using a Neo-Hookean material was exported to

Abaqus. Finally, MSML was used to color the meshes for visualization purposes and to quantitatively compare the real-time algorithm with the Abaqus ground truth model.

```
<mesh>
 <quadraticTetMesh name="liverMesh" filename="
     @meshConverter" >
  <tet10MeshConverter name="meshConverter"
  quadraticMesh="liverVolumeTet10Mesh.vtk" linearMesh="
      @liverVolumeMesher" />
  <mesherTetgen name="liverVolumeMesher" mesh="
      liverVolumeMesh.vtk"
  surfaceMesh="@meshReducer" preserveBoundary = "1" />
  <meshReductionOperator name="meshReducer" outputMesh="
      liverXSSurface.vtk"
  inputMesh="liverSurface.vtk" numberOfTriangles = "200" />
 </quadraticTetMesh>
</mesh>
```

Figure 9.2.: MSML operator chain to convert a high resolution surface mesh to a low-resolution quadratic tetrahedral FE mesh.

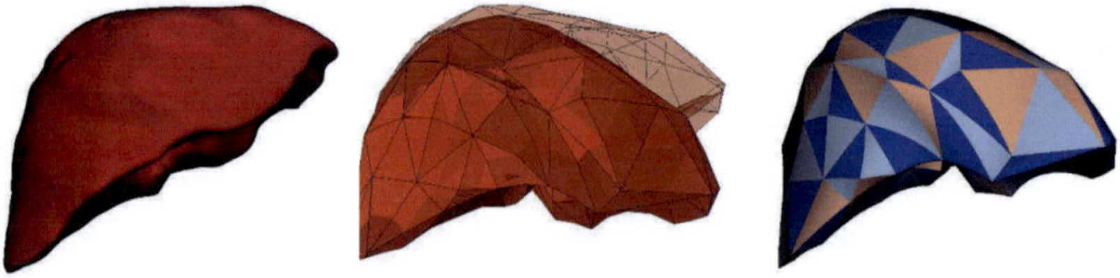

Figure 9.3.: Quadratic tetrahedral finite element meshes were automatically built from a high-resolution surface mesh (left) and solved using a real-time corotated algorithm within the SOFA framework (middle) and fully non-linear Neo-Hookean model within the ABAQUS FE-package (right).

Multi organ simulation for radio therapy

In the framework of the Collaborative Research Centre *Cognition Guided Surgery*, the MSML was adapted by Stoll et al. to simulate organ motion for radiation therapy planning. In this context a multi organ model was constructed from a segmented torso dataset from the Ircad database [2] (Fig. 9.4). The MSML was used to create the volume mesh, to define the mechanical material parameters as well as the boundary conditions. The simulation was performed using the SOFA simulation framework [FDD+12].

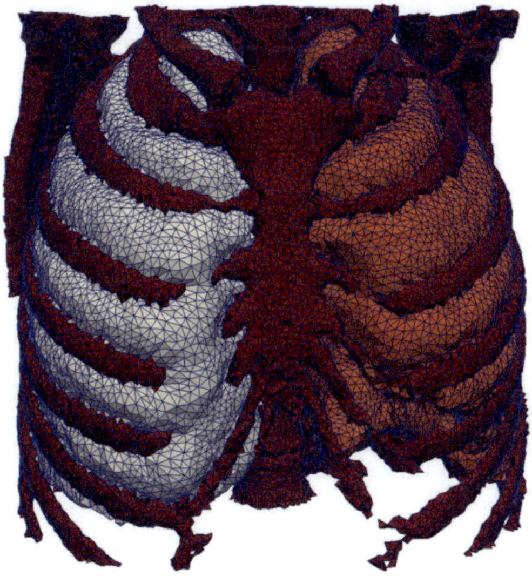

Figure 9.4.: A pressure boundary condition is applied to the inner surfaces of both lungs (from [SSS+14]).

9.1.4. Towards intuitive finite element based simulations

The Medical Simulation Markup Language acts as a middleware between all tools used in the biomechanical modeling pipeline. This

[2] www.ircad.fr/softwares/3Dircadb

allows to quickly set-up biomechanical modeling workflows for development, prototyping and system validation. The unique feature of the approach is its flexibility; new components, operators or material types can be added by simply providing an XML-based description. The Python based implementation is available as open-source software from github.com/CognitionGuidedSurgery/msml. More material models, operators and exporters (e.g. to FEBio) are continuously integrate into the framework.
Even with a tool like MSML available, a lot of expert knowledge is required to set-up biomedical simulations. Suitable modeling techniques and material models have to be selected in order to simulate the mechanical behavior of different anatomical objects and physiological processes. Furthermore, numerical expertise is required to choose suitable algorithms and solvers for each problem. In typical mechanical engineering applications for computer aided engineering (e.g. automotive, aerospace) there are specially trained analysts that set up the numerical simulations for the design engineers.
We are currently working on integrating a cognitive assistance into MSML that can play the role of the simulation analyst and can help to make elaborate simulation technology available for non-experts. In this context we are using ontologies in order to encapsulate the necessary explicit background knowledge. In addition, machine learning techniques are used for automatic parameter selection (e.g. for volumetric grid generation). We believe that an intuitive biomechanical workflow is essential for establishing simulations techniques in the clinical workflow.

9.2. Validating and benchmarking CAS systems

Determining the accuracy of computer assisted surgery (CAS) systems is challenging [JGMJ06]. This is in particular true in the realm of minimally invasive soft tissue interventions. Here, it is very complicated and sometimes even impossible to obtain reliable *in vivo* ground truth data. In this section, a novel approach for manufacturing mechanically accurate soft tissue phantoms is presented. Furthermore, numerics (*in silico*) based validation strategies are discussed and we introduce Open-CAS, a web platform for open data in the context of CAS validation.

9.2.1. Mechanically accurate soft tissue phantoms

Organ phantoms are a popular approach to validating algorithms for image guided surgery. In contrast to animal experiments, phantom based validation is cheap, repeatable and often allows determining ground truth data with a lot less post-processing. In this context, silicone is a promising phantom material as it is chemically robust and retains its mechanical characteristics for years. However, it is very challenging to produce silicone phantoms whose mechanical response really mimics biological soft tissue. In the following we present an approach to manufacture accurate soft tissue phantoms and show how these can be used to build multi-organ phantoms.

Silicones for soft tissue mimicking phantoms

Most industrially used silicones are much stiffer than biological soft tissue. Adding a so called *slacker* component is one possibility to soften these materials. However, silicones that are softened in this way usually have a very tacky surface, which makes processing difficult. Silicone models are typically cast from two different fluid components. Upon contact these components trigger a crosslink of the raw materials which then cure to the final product in a couple of hours. In some cases it is possible to control the stiffness of the silicone by changing the ratio in which the components are mixed together.
Based on the stiffness requirements for soft tissue phantoms, several groups of silicones from different vendors were evaluated with respect to their application for organ phantoms: Wacker Silgel 612, Wacker Elastosil 7616-195, Wacker Elastosil P26028, Kaupo DragonSkin, Kaupo EcoFlex10 and Kaupo EcoFlex30. In cooperation with the Institute for Technical Chemistry and Polymer Chemistry at the Karlsruhe Institute of Technology, these silicones where analyzed within an Eplexor rheometer (Fig. 9.5).
During the rheometrical analysis, each sample was compressed by 40%. Based on the forces that were measured during each compression step, the Young modulus of each material was then calculated for the different load points (Fig. 9.6). We also performed a literature review in order to extract relevant material parameters that have been determined by other groups for different organs such as the liver or the prostate. Suitable

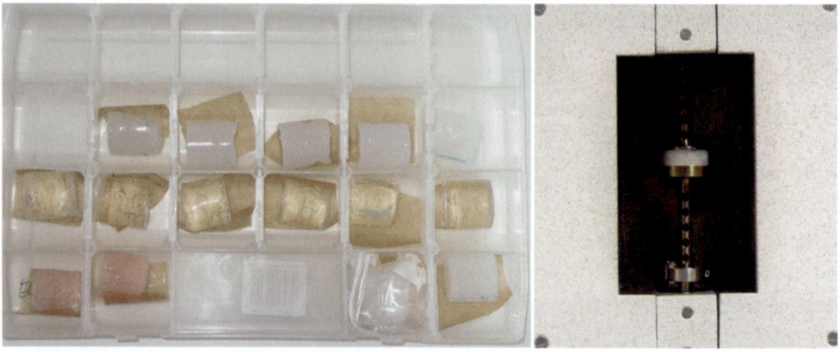

Figure 9.5.: A sample was manufactured from several silicone mixtures (left) which were subsequently analyzed using an Eplexor rheometer (right).

silicones were then selected based on the measurements, the models obtained from the literature and other properties that are important for manufacturing (e.g. tackiness, tear-resistance). For the liver, Elastosil P26038 proved to be an ideal candidate due to its low stiffness and smooth surface properties.

Manufacturing silicone based abdominal organs

In order to build a silicone liver phantom, a human liver was segmented from CT images (Fig. 9.7). A CAD model of the phantom molds was subsequently constructed from the liver surface model using the Materialise 3Matic software package. The design of the molds was optimized with respect to cheap rapid prototyping. The liver phantom was finally cast from the printed molds (Fig. 9.8) in different layers. This allowed inserting a regular pattern of small Teflon marker balls (diameter of 3.175mm) into the phantom for accurate tracking of the deformation field in CT images.
A complete torso phantom was designed at the University Hospital Heidelberg using the presented manufacturing techniques. The design is completely based on segmented CT images. A rigid outline of the body as well as bony structures were also manufactured using rapid prototyping techniques (Fig. 9.9). OpenHELP allows simulating more complex

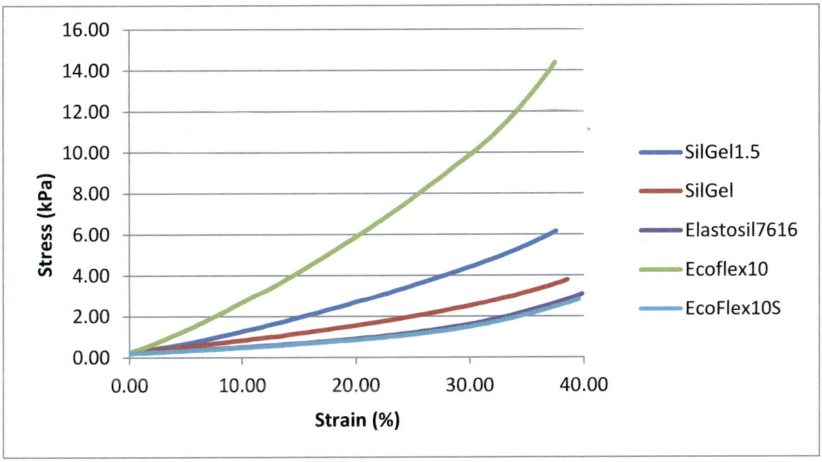

Figure 9.6.: Young's modulus in kPa in terms of compressive strain for selected silicones.

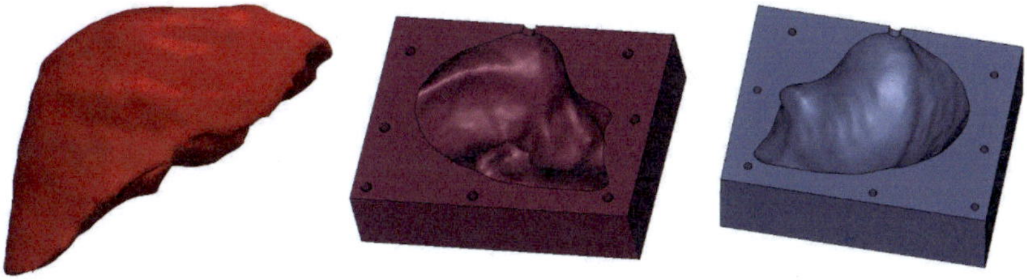

Figure 9.7.: Liver surface model obtained from segmented CT images (left) and CAD models of phantom molds (middle, right).

deformation pattern and inter-organ interaction. As all deformations can be easily tracked in CT images thanks to the markers in the silicone organs, the model thus serves as a very useful validation tool for CAS components. It even offers a cheap, reproducible and accurate alternative to animal experiments for many validation steps. A sample application for the validation of 3D stereo reconstruction algorithms from endoscopic data is shown in Fig. 9.9.

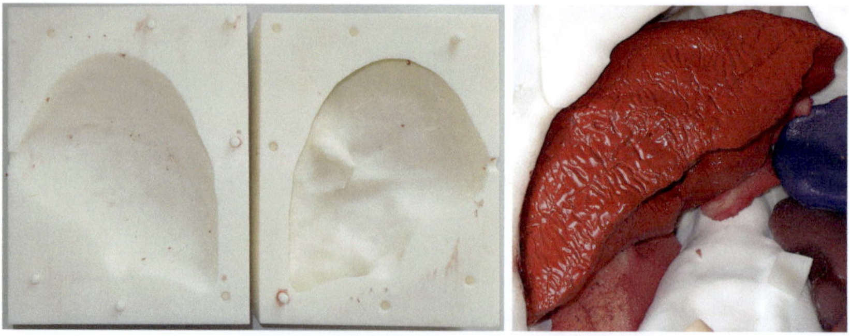

Figure 9.8.: Upper and lower casting mold manufactured using rapid prototyping techniques (left, middle) and final silicone liver inside the OpenHELP torso phantom (right).

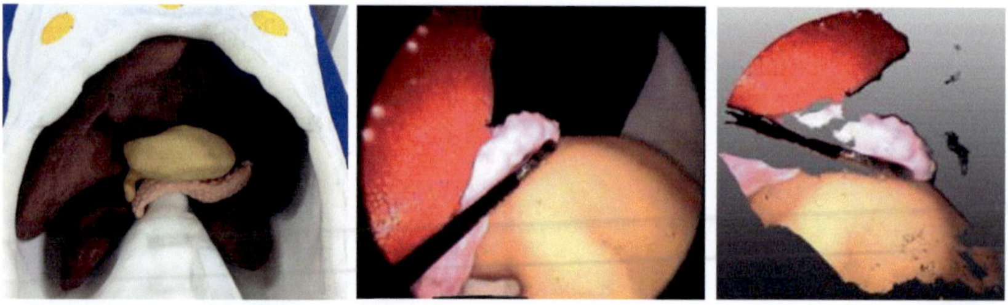

Figure 9.9.: OpenHELP torso phantom built from segmented CT images (left), endoscopic video frame featuring several silicone organs (middle) and corresponding 3D-reconstruction from stereo endoscopic data (right).

Phantoms with non-linear response

It can be seen from Fig. 9.6 that most silicones exhibit a very linear behavior even in the presence of large strains. In contrast, the mechanical behavior of biological soft tissues is strongly non-linear. One possibility to mimic real tissue behavior over a larger deformation range, the phantoms can be equipped with a stiff core and a softer outer region (Fig. 9.10).
In this setup the question naturally arise how the parameters of the phantom (e.g. stiffness and size of the core, stiffness of the outer shell)

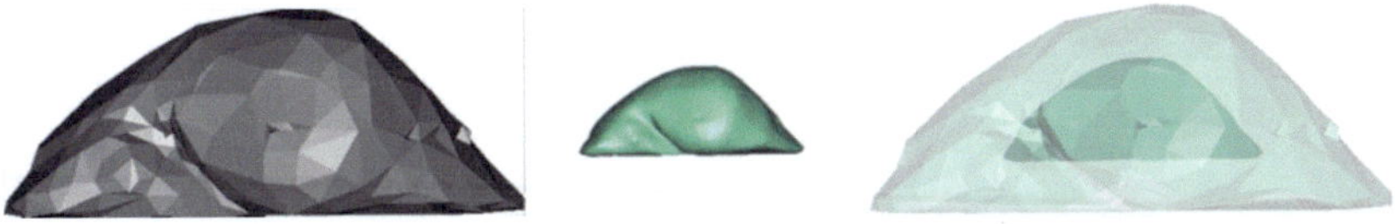

Figure 9.10.: On order to achieve a strongly non-linear mechanical response, the organ phantom is equipped with a stiff core and a softer outer region.

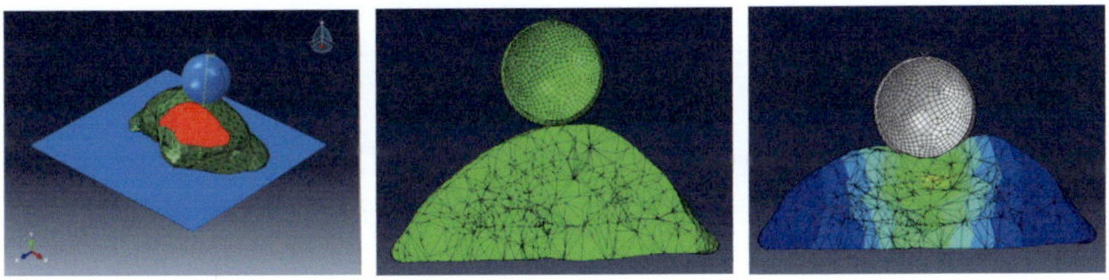

Figure 9.11.: Model of an indentation experiment in Abaqus (left). Initial (undeformed) configuration (middle) and deformed configuration with color-coded von Mises stress (right).

should be determined. In order to address this problem we developed a prototypical optimization approach for identifying these parameters. For this purpose we model an indentation on the organ phantom with the Abaqus FE package (Fig. 9.11). We use a Levenberg-Marquardt optimization scheme and approximate the Jacobian by using a finite difference scheme on the Abaqus-based forward FE simulation. This parameter identification procedure is able to find suitable stiffness parameters for the core and the shell for a fixed core size. In the future, the scheme will be extended towards analyzing multiple load conditions (not just a single indentation) and a variable core size. However, this scenario is challenging as the optimization problem does not have a unique solution and the can thus easily be easily trapped in local minima.

Workflow for *ground truth* computation

Evaluating phantom validation experiments is usually a very time-consuming task. First, organs of interest have to be segmented. We

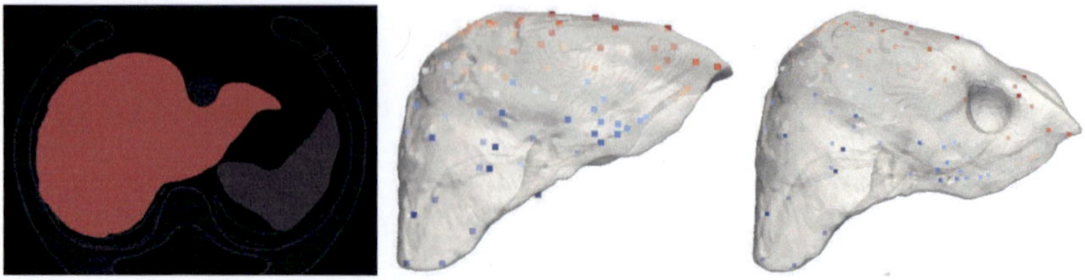

Figure 9.12.: Post-processing of a phantom validation experiment involves semi-automatic segmentation of relevant organs (left) and automatic extraction of marker displacements for different deformation states (middle, right).

use snake-based algorithms implemented in the open source ITK-SNAP[3] toolkit to perform this procedure in a semi-automatic way (Fig. 9.12). A fully automatic algorithm was developed in order to segment all Teflon marker balls and perform a registration between different states of deformation: Due to the size and density of the marker balls, the segmentation can be performed using a simple threshold procedure. Afterwards all connected regions in the image are labeled and all regions whose pixel size is smaller than a certain threshold are discarded. The center for each of the marker balls is then determined by computing the center of mass for each blob. In this way, a point cloud is extracted for each deformation state.

In order to obtain a ground truth deformation, these point clouds have to be registered for every deformation state. This is challenging as artefacts in the CT images often cause the segmentation procedure to produce point clouds of different sizes for each deformation state. Therefore, straight forward approaches to tackle the registration problem such as a nearest neighbor search are unreliable. Instead, we use the previously mentioned coherent point drift (CPD) algorithm to perform the registration in a stable way. Due to the added regularization in the algorithm, the point clouds are accurately registered and it is easy to verify if marker points are lost or added between different states of deformation.

[3]www.itksnap.org

9.2.2. *in silico* evaluation suite

It has already become apparent throughout this thesis (especially in chapter 7) that the numerical computation of ground truth data (*in silico* validation) is an important technique for the validation of research prototypes in the area of computer assisted surgery. This approach allows obtaining dense ground truth data in a reliable and repeatable way.
Röhl et al. presented a simulation environment for accuracy validation of 3D reconstruction techniques for stereo endoscopes [RBS+12]. Based on an accurate camera model, the tool uses realistic organ textures and appropriate lighting models in order to reproduce the optical properties commonly found in endoscopic image sequences (e.g. specular reflections). It generates all necessary ground truth data such as the disparity map of the 3D scene (see Fig. 9.13).
Current work aims at including more sensor data into the simulation tool (e.g. tracking information). Furthermore, a soft tissue simulation based on a corotated FE technique is integrated into the tool. This allows validating image processing and registration algorithms in the presence of physically realistic soft tissue deformations.
In order to enhance the realism of such a simulation tool for laparoscopic interventions, a suitable user interface is necessary. For this reason, high-fidelity haptic interfaces have become an important part of VR simulators for minimally invasive surgery (MIS) training [CMJ11]. However, the availability of these devices for validation purposes in CAS research is severely limited due to the high costs of this special purpose hardware. In order to overcome this obstacle we have developed a low-cost laparoscopic haptic input device based on the Novint Falcon game controller (Fig. 9.14).
The customizations such as the special grip for the Falcon are manufactured using rapid prototyping techniques. In addition the device can be assembled without specific tools (with exception of the sensor circuit board). The total cost of 1800 Euro is very low compared to standard equipment. Further development aims at making the hardware design along with the necessary software drivers available under an open source license. For more information on the project we refer to the corresponding publication [SRB+14].

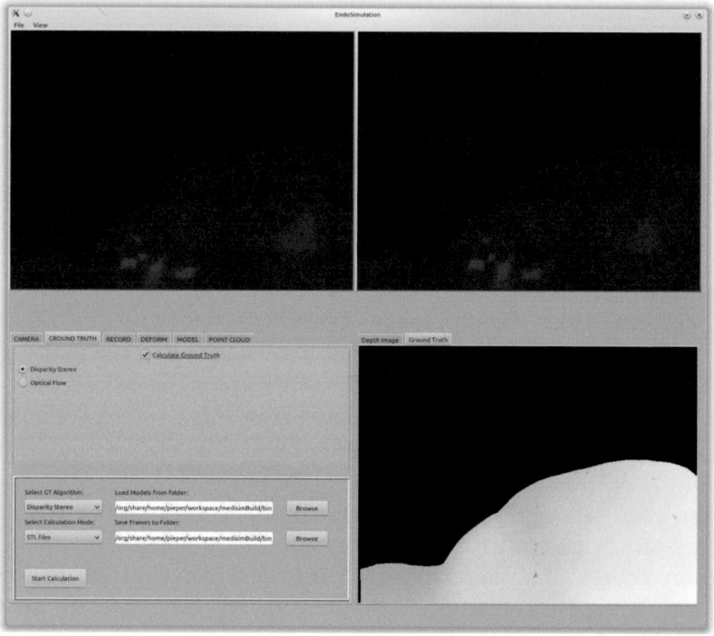

Figure 9.13.: A simulation environment allows to compute accurate *ground truth* data such as the disparity ground truth between the left and right stereo image or depth maps.

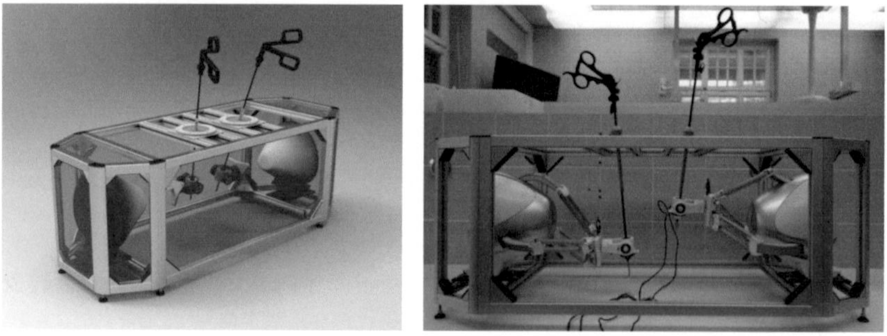

Figure 9.14.: CAD design (left) and prototype (right) of a low-cost laparoscopic input device (from [SRB+14])

9.2.3. Open-Cas: Towards open data for CAS validation

Regardless if using *in silico* evaluation, soft tissue phantoms or animal experiments, the design of reliable validation experiments is non-trivial and time consuming. Furthermore, the execution and post processing of experimental results from phantom or animal experiments require not only the access to CT imaging hardware, but also manual effort (e.g. segmentation).
Having common data sets does not only allow researchers to spend more time on development and less time on validation, but it also allows to benchmark algorithms against each other. In the realm of computer vision, the Middlebury datasets are widely used for that purpose [SS02]. Although there are some datasets for the validation of CAS components available (e.g. the Hamlyn Centre endoscopic video datasets [SSPY10] and the 3D-IRCAD database [3Di13]), it would be desirable to have a more extensive selection of data. In particular, it would be beneficial to establish a common repository that can serve not only as a central access point for data, but also for benchmark results. As the complexity of the data is growing (e.g. different types of temporally registered sensor data) it is especially important to develop standardized data formats and corresponding processing tools in order to make the data easily accessible.
Naturally, such a repository should not be limited to numerical or phantom data. In the context of image processing (e.g. instrument segmentation) *in vivo* sensor data is often used for qualitative evaluation. In some contexts, manually labeled image data can even serve as a reliable ground truth. Making these kinds of data freely available would significantly speed up the development for many research groups. This is even more true for algorithms that rely on machine learning approaches such as segmentation or situation recognition techniques [KWG+13a]. In these applications, the acquisition and manual processing of suitable learning and test data often is the most time consuming part of development.
The website Open-Cas.org (Fig. 9.15) is a first attempt at establishing a platform for open data in the context of CAS validation [SRB+13]. Currently, both numerical and phantom based validation data is available on the platform. More validation data is continuously added to the database.

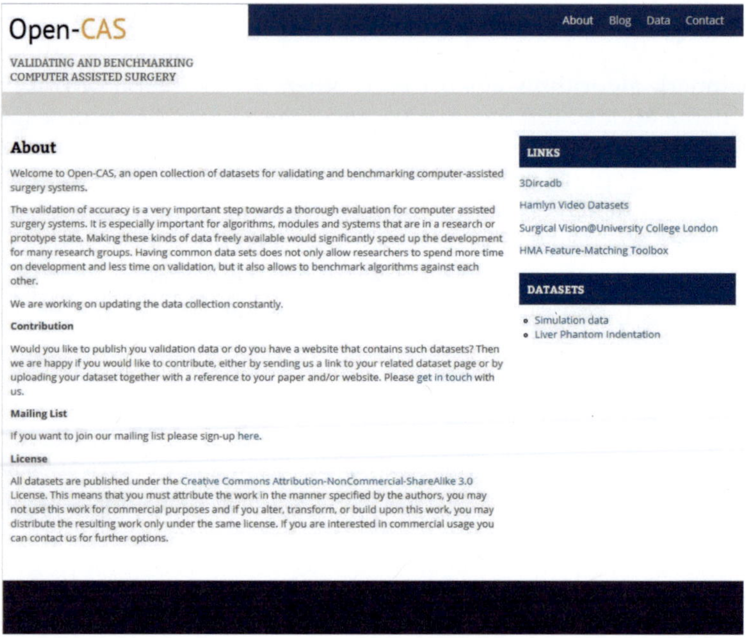

Figure 9.15.: The Open-CAS website is a publication platform for open data in the context of CAS validation [SRB$^+$13].

Prediction is very difficult, especially about the future.

— Niels Bohr

10. Conclusions

Computer assisted surgery (CAS) systems intraoperatively support the surgeon by providing information on the location of hidden risk (e.g. vessels, nerves) and target structures (e.g. tumors) during surgery. In this way CAS techniques have been a major driving force for improving patient outcomes for many applications such as orthopedic surgery and neurosurgery. However, CAS is currently not used in the daily clinical routine for laparoscopic interventions. The main reason for this discrepancy are soft tissue deformations that make intraoperative registration (and thus intraoperative navigation) difficult. In this work, a novel, biomechanics based approach for real-time soft tissue registration from sparse intraoperative sensor data such as stereo endoscopic images was researched. In the upcoming section, we sum up the methods that have been developed in this context. The discussion will be guided by the research questions that have been outlined at the beginning of this thesis (section 1.1). In addition, further research paths that build on the results of this work are highlighted.

10.1. Summary

The main purpose of this work was to develop a novel approach for soft tissue registration in the context of laparoscopic partial liver resection. At the core of the approach lies an accurate, yet real-time capable finite element (FE) model of the liver. A novel GPU-based FE solver allows to efficiently solve even large models in real-time. During the novel physics-based registration process, this biomechanical model serves as a regularization term in order to match a preoperative model to an intraoperative surface geometry. The results and contributions of this thesis can be summarized as follows:

- **Real-time biomechanical model for soft tissue registration**
  By means of a thorough simulation study it was shown that the registration accuracy does only depend very weakly on the material model type and its parameterization. Based in this insight a **corotated elasticity model** was presented for efficient, yet accurate soft tissue registration. The numerical efficiency of this model was greatly enhanced through several new algorithms. First, it was demonstrated that isoparametric quadratic tetrahedral elements are superior to linear tetrahedral grids for soft tissue simulation. In order to leverage the potential of quadratic elements in a real-time setting, a novel scheme for **accurately embedding high resolution surfaces into higher order elements** was developed. We also presented a novel **GPU based multigrid finite element solver** that further speeds up the simulation. The developed multigrid approach for solving elasticity problems is unique for two reasons. It is not only the **first multigrid scheme for solving elasticity problems on unstructured, non-conforming, higher order grids**, but also the first approach to a **GPU-based multigrid solver for the real-time simulation of deformable models on unstructured grids**. In this context, the aforementioned novel mapping was used in order to transfer displacements and forces between the meshes in the grid hierarchy. In order to achieve high efficiency on parallel hardware, a sparse approximate inverse approach was used for preconditioning and smoothing. In order to make this operator real-time capable, it is pre-computed and subsequently adapted to the current deformation each time step (*rotation warping*). In contrast to the state-of-the-art (using linear tetrahedral grids and a Jacobi-preconditioned CG solver), the novel method can achieve speedups of several orders of magnitude.

- **Physics based shape matching for stable real-time soft tissue registration in the context of laparoscopic liver resection**
  As an important use case for soft tissue registration in laparoscopic surgery, a system for registering preoperative planning data to intraoperative stereo endoscopic image data in the context of partial liver resection was developed. Here, a 3D surface model of the

surgical site was obtained through 3D reconstruction of the stereo endoscopic video data and image stitching. In order to match the preoperative organ model to an intraoperative partial surface, we presented the novel **physics based shape matching** (PBSM) scheme. This approach treats the non-rigid surface registration as an electrostatic-elastic problem, where an elastic body that is electrically charged (preoperative model) slides into an oppositely charged rigid shape (intraoperative surface). In contrast to previous attempts at biomechanically based registration, this novel physics based interpretation allows casting the shape matching problem into a single variational formulation. It is also the first method that employs a non-linear, yet real-time capable biomechanical model of the liver for registration purposes. As the technique is based on a preoperative volumetric FE model, it naturally recovers the position of volumetric structures (e.g. tumors or vessels). In a large validation study based on numerical and phantom data, it was shown that the **novel method severely outperforms the state-of-the-art** *coherent point drift* algorithm. It can be concluded from this analysis that **biomechanically based regularization by means of corotated elasticity is a highly promising strategy** for soft tissue registration based on sparse intraoperative sensor data. Furthermore, it was shown how known landmark correspondence (e.g. through texture or ultrasound tracking) can be integrated into the PBSM scheme and the algorithm was integrated into the MediAssist CAS system.

- **Finite element methods for flexible discontinuity and geometry embedding**
  The topology of the surgical site changes due to tissue cutting during many interventions (e.g. partial liver resection). This poses a big challenge for finite element based biomechanical models as online re-meshing of the topology changes can severely impair the performance and the stability of the simulation. In this work, we analyzed an alternative approach for modeling discontinuities in the solution by enriching the affected elements with special shape functions. In particular, we showed how so called extended FEM (X-FEM) techniques can be used to **simulate arbitrary cuts through corotated elastic models**. Furthermore, it was shown how the discontinuous Galerkin (DG-FEM) method can be used for

an efficient embedding of the enriched elements. The performed validation studies demonstrate that these techniques are superior to re-meshing approaches in terms of stability and accuracy per degrees of freedom.

- **Intuitive biomechanical model workflow**
In the course of this thesis work, it became apparent that the construction of patient-specific biomechanical models from tomographic data is a non-trivial workflow and time consuming task. Although a diverse ecosystem of software tools exists for each of step of this workflow, there was no solution that allowed combining and accessing these tools in an intuitive and easy way. This problem is also highly relevant in other research areas that make use of biomechanical models such as diagnostics (e.g. for cardiovascular diseases), intervention planning and training. It can even be argued that the lack of **intuitive software tools** for the construction of patient-specific biomechanical models is a major barrier for a widespread adoption of these procedures into clinical research. In order to overcome this problem, the flexible XML-based **Medical Simulation Markup Language (MSML)** was proposed, implemented and made available as open-source software.

- **Validation tools for CAS**
Accuracy validation of CAS systems is challenging. In the realm of minimally invasive visceral interventions, it is very complicated and sometimes even impossible to obtain reliable *in vivo* ground truth data. In this work we presented several novel tools for CAS validation. Most importantly, an approach for manufacturing **mechanically accurate silicone soft tissue phantoms** was developed. Through the course of the validation experiments for the PBSM scheme it was shown how small marker balls inside these organ models can be used to track deformations in CT imaging. In addition to phantom based experiments, we also discussed numerics (*in silico*) based validation strategies and introduced **Open-CAS.org, a web platform for open data** in the context of CAS validation. These methods not only help to reduce the number of necessary animal experiments and help researchers to spend more time on algorithm development and less time on validation. They also open

up the path for establishing benchmark datasets in the realm of computer assisted surgery.

10.2. Outlook

No scientific work is ever complete, but rather opens up new avenues for further research. For the methods presented in this thesis, additional work should in particular focus on translating the developed techniques towards the clinical setting. In addition to smaller implementation related issues such as improving data structures to enhance the numerical efficiency or implementing a GPU version of the PBSM scheme, four interesting areas for further work can be identified. These will be briefly discussed in this section.

- **Validation of the PBSM approach through animal experiments**
  The accuracy of the developed physics based shape matching (PBSM) scheme has already been extensively validated using numerical data and phantom experiments. Validating the approach in the context of a porcine partial liver resection is the next step towards demonstrating its clinical viability. In this context it will be especially interesting to see, if the internal vessel structure of the liver (that has not been modeled in this work) has a noticeable effect on the registration accuracy. Furthermore, the performance of the system should be evaluated in the presence of strong pathologies (e.g. cirrhosis of the liver). The design of such an *in vivo* validation experiment has to be carefully planned in order to obtain reliable ground truth data. On option might be to perfuse the liver with contrast agent in order to track the deformation of vessel bifurcations in CT images. Currently, there is no publicly available data for these kinds of experiments. Thus, we plan to release the data from such an animal validation experiment under an open license on Open-CAS.org in order to help validating and benchmarking a wide variety of algorithms in the domain of registration and image processing for CAS.

- **Inter-organ interactions and estimating boundary conditions on hidden surfaces**
  Within the PBSM validation experiments, we used a very simple

model for the boundary conditions (BC) on the hidden surfaces and either assumed zero force or zero displacement BC on different parts of the liver. In order to further enhance the accuracy of the PBSM scheme, it is necessary to introduce more complex models of these boundary conditions. One possibility is to not only consider a single organ in the biomechanical model, but to build a multi-organ model that accurately simulates the organ-interactions on the hidden surfaces. However, such a model is not only computationally intensive, but also difficult to build and to parameterize for each patient. A better option might be to use additional ultrasound imaging to extract volumetric landmarks. By using an optimization scheme on top of the PBSM approach, the boundary conditions on the hidden surfaces can then be estimated from these landmarks.

- **Hierarchical non-boundary fitting discretizations**
  Techniques that evolve around the analyzed DG-FEM and X-FEM ultimately allow efficiently simulating problems with meshes that do not resemble the actual geometry. This helps to remove the difficult meshing step in the biomechanical simulation workflow. Furthermore it makes constructing model hierarchies easy and thus allow for a straight forward implementation of multigrid solvers. The approach can be especially beneficial to solve biomechanical problems on massive parallel hardware. First of all, these techniques allow the use of structured, rectangular grids that result in data structures that are well suited for GPU based computations. Furthermore, the necessary model representations and data structure for such a biomechanical model can be directly derived from segmented tomographic images.

- **Intuitive workflows for patient-specific biomechanical models**
  A lot of expert knowledge is required in order to build a biomechanical model from segmented tomographic images: Suitable modeling techniques and material models have to be selected in order to simulate the mechanical behavior of different anatomical objects and physiological processes. Furthermore, numerical expertise is required to choose suitable algorithms and solvers for each problem. Even with a tool like the Medical Simulation Markup Language available, this complexity will still hinder the translation of biomechanically based methods into clinical research. That is

why we are currently working towards a cognitive assistance that encapsulates the knowledge of experienced simulation analysts and can help to make elaborate simulation technology available for non-experts. In this context we are using ontologies in order to encapsulate the necessary explicit background knowledge. In addition, machine learning techniques are used for automatic parameter selection (e.g. for volumetric grid generation).

A.

Additional remarks on elasticity theory and FE methods

A.1. Basics of vector analysis

A.1.1. Divergence theorem

For any smooth vector field $\mathbf{v}(\mathbf{x})$ and any smooth tensor field $\mathbf{A}(\mathbf{x})$ that are defined on a compact region Ω which is enclosed by the smooth, closed surface $\partial\Omega$ we have

$$\int_{\partial\Omega} \mathbf{v} \cdot \mathbf{n} \mathrm{dA} = \int_{\Omega} \mathrm{div}\mathbf{v} \mathrm{dV} \qquad \text{or} \qquad \int_{\partial\Omega} v_i n_i \mathrm{dA} = \int_{\Omega} \frac{\partial v_i}{\partial x_i} \mathrm{dV} \tag{A.1}$$

$$\int_{\partial\Omega} \mathbf{A}\mathbf{n} \mathrm{dA} = \int_{\Omega} \mathrm{div}\mathbf{A} \mathrm{dV} \qquad \text{or} \qquad \int_{\partial\Omega} A_{ij} n_j \mathrm{dA} = \int_{\Omega} \frac{\partial A_{ij}}{\partial x_j} \mathrm{dV} \tag{A.2}$$

A.1.2. Product differentiation rules for tensors

For any smooth vector field $\mathbf{v}(\mathbf{x})$ and any smooth tensor field $\mathbf{A}(\mathbf{x})$ we have

$$\mathrm{div}(\mathbf{A}^T\mathbf{v}) = \mathrm{div}(\mathbf{A}) \cdot \mathbf{v} + \mathrm{div}(\mathbf{A}) : \mathrm{grad}(\mathbf{v}) \tag{A.3}$$

A.2. Work conjugancy of S and $\dot{\mathrm{E}}$

It has already been shown in section (4.2.1) that the first Piola-Kirchhoff stress tensor $\mathbf{P}$ is work conjugated to the material time derivative of the deformation gradient **F**. It is quickly shown that the material time derivative of the Cauchy-Green strain tensor **C**

$$\dot{\mathbf{C}} = \frac{\mathrm{D}}{\mathrm{D}t}\left(\mathbf{F}^T\mathbf{F}\right) = \dot{\mathbf{F}}^T\mathbf{F} + \mathbf{F}^T\dot{\mathbf{F}} \tag{A.4}$$

related to the material time derivative of the Green-Lagrange strain tensor by

$$\dot{\mathbf{E}} = \frac{\mathrm{D}}{\mathrm{D}t}\frac{1}{2}\left(\mathbf{F}^T\mathbf{F} - \mathbf{I}\right) = \frac{1}{2}\left(\dot{\mathbf{F}}^T\mathbf{F} + \mathbf{F}^T\dot{\mathbf{F}}\right) = \frac{1}{2}\dot{\mathbf{C}}. \tag{A.5}$$

Based on the results of section 4.2.1 (work conjugancy of **P** and $\dot{\mathbf{F}}$), we can thus derive

$$\mathbf{P} : \dot{\mathbf{F}} = \mathrm{tr}(\mathbf{P}^T\dot{\mathbf{F}}) = \mathrm{tr}(\dot{\mathbf{F}}^T\mathbf{P}) = \mathrm{tr}(\dot{\mathbf{F}}^T\mathbf{F}\underbrace{\mathbf{F}^{-1}\mathbf{P}}_{\mathbf{S}}) \tag{A.6}$$

$$= \mathrm{tr}(\mathbf{S}\dot{\mathbf{F}}^T\mathbf{F}) = \mathrm{tr}(\mathbf{S}\mathbf{F}\dot{\mathbf{F}}^T) = \mathrm{tr}(\mathbf{S}\frac{1}{2}(\dot{\mathbf{F}}^T\mathbf{F} + \mathbf{F}\dot{\mathbf{F}}^T)) \tag{A.7}$$

$$= \frac{1}{2}\mathbf{S} : \dot{\mathbf{C}} = \mathbf{S} : \dot{\mathbf{E}} \tag{A.8}$$

A.3. The Saint Venant-Kirchhoff model

The elastic energy functional for Saint-Venant Kirchhoff model is defined by

$$\Psi(\mathbf{E}) = \frac{\lambda}{2}(\mathrm{tr}\mathbf{E})^2 + \mu\mathrm{tr}(\mathbf{E}^2). \tag{A.9}$$

In order to express the relation

$$\mathbf{S}(\mathbf{E}) = \frac{\partial\Psi(\mathbf{E})}{\partial\mathbf{E}}, \tag{A.10}$$

we note the partial derivatives

$$\frac{\partial\mathrm{tr}(\mathbf{E})}{\partial\mathbf{E}} = \frac{1}{\partial E_{ij}}\sum_{k=1}^{3} E_{kk} = \delta_{ij} = \mathbf{I} \tag{A.11}$$

and

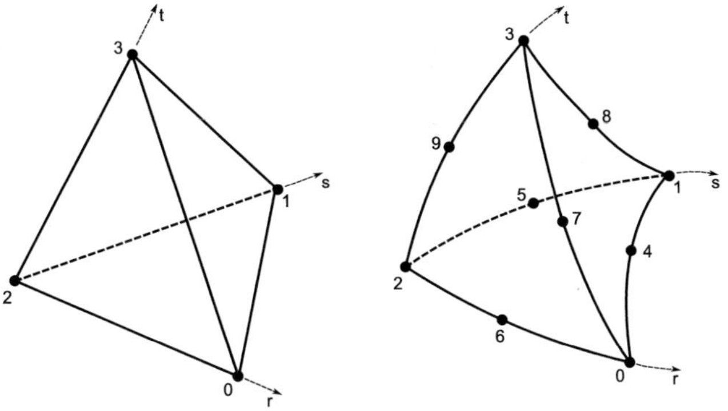

Figure A.1.: Linear tetrahedron with 4 nodes (tet4) and quadratic tetrahedron with 10 nodes (tet10)

$$\mathbf{S}(\partial\mathbf{E}) = \frac{\partial \mathrm{tr}(\mathbf{E}^2)}{\partial \mathbf{E}} = \frac{1}{\partial E_{ij}} \sum_{k,l=1}^{3} E_{kl}E_{kl} = 2E_{ij} = 2\mathbf{E}. \tag{A.12}$$

Thus, we obtain

$$\frac{\partial\Psi(\mathbf{E})}{\partial\mathbf{E}} = \frac{\lambda}{2}\frac{\partial\left((\mathrm{tr}\mathbf{E})^2\right)}{\partial\mathbf{E}} + \mu\frac{\partial\left(\mathrm{tr}(\mathbf{E}^2)\right)}{\partial\mathbf{E}} = \lambda\mathrm{tr}\mathbf{E}\mathbf{I} + 2\mu\mathbf{E}. \tag{A.13}$$

A.4. Polynomial shape functions for selected elements

A.4.1. Nodal shape functions in local (curvilinear) coordinates

Linear 4-node tetrahedron (node numbering as shown in Fig. A.1):

$$N_0(r,s,t) = r \tag{A.14}$$
$$N_2(r,s,t) = s \tag{A.15}$$
$$N_3(r,s,t) = 1 - r - s - t \tag{A.16}$$
$$N_4(r,s,t) = t \tag{A.17}$$
(A.18)

Quadratic 10-node tetrahedron (node numbering as shown in Fig. A.1):

$$N_0(r,s,t) = (2r-1)r \tag{A.19}$$
$$N_1(r,s,t) = (2s-1)s \tag{A.20}$$
$$N_2(r,s,t) = (2(1-r-s-t)-1)(1-r-s-t) \tag{A.21}$$
$$N_3(r,s,t) = (2t-1)t \tag{A.22}$$
$$N_4(r,s,t) = 4rs \tag{A.23}$$
$$N_5(r,s,t) = 4(1-r-s-t)s \tag{A.24}$$
$$N_6(r,s,t) = 4(1-r-s-t)r \tag{A.25}$$
$$N_7(r,s,t) = 4st \tag{A.26}$$
$$N_8(r,s,t) = 4rt \tag{A.27}$$
$$N_9(r,s,t) = 4(1-r-s-t)t \tag{A.28}$$
(A.29)

A.4.2. Nodal shape functions in global coordinates

The standard triangle [(1,0,0) (0,1,0) (0,0,0) (0,0,1)] is mapped to the global coordinate system using the shape functions (isometric elements). If $\mathbf{X}_k$ denotes the initial position of the k-th node of the n-node tetrahedron, we define the function $\xi(\mathbf{r})$ that maps the local coordinates $\mathbf{r} = (r,s,t)$ to the global coordinates $\mathbf{X} = (X_1, X_2, X_3)$:

$$\xi(\mathbf{r}) = \mathbf{X}(\mathbf{r}) = \mathbf{X}(r,s,t) = \sum_{k=0}^{n} \mathbf{X}_k N_k(r,s,t) \tag{A.30}$$

The global derivatives of the shape functions are

$$\frac{\partial N_I(\mathbf{x})}{\partial \mathbf{X}} = \mathbf{J}^{-1} \frac{\partial N_I(\mathbf{x})}{\partial \mathbf{r}} \tag{A.31}$$

where $\mathbf{J}$ is the jacobian

$$\mathbf{J} = \nabla \xi = \begin{pmatrix} \frac{\partial X_1}{\partial r} & \frac{\partial X_2}{\partial r} & \frac{\partial X_3}{\partial r} \\ \frac{\partial X_1}{\partial s} & \frac{\partial X_2}{\partial s} & \frac{\partial X_3}{\partial s} \\ \frac{\partial X_1}{\partial t} & \frac{\partial X_2}{\partial t} & \frac{\partial X_3}{\partial t} \end{pmatrix} \tag{A.32}$$

A.5. Internal nodal forces and the stiffness matrix for linear elasticity

As detailed in section 5.2.1, the internal nodal forces are given by

$$\mathbf{f}^{int} = f_{iI}^{int} = \int_{\Omega_0} \hat{f}_{iI}^{X,int} \mathrm{dV}_0 = \sum_e \int_\tau \hat{f}_{iI}^{X,int} \mathrm{dV}_0 = \int_{\Omega_0} \sigma_{ik} (\nabla N)_{kI} \mathrm{dV}_0 \tag{A.33}$$

By noting that the gradient of the displacement vector reads

$$\nabla \mathbf{u} = \nabla(\mathcal{U}_I N_I) = \mathcal{U}_I \nabla N_I = \mathcal{U}_{iI} (\nabla N)_{kI}, \tag{A.34}$$

we can express its the derivative with respect to the nodal displacements through

$$\frac{\partial}{\partial \mathcal{U}_{jJ}} (\nabla \mathcal{U})_{ik} = \frac{\partial}{\partial \mathcal{U}_{jJ}} (\mathcal{U}_{iI} (\nabla N)_{kI}) = \delta_{ij} (\nabla N_{kJ}). \tag{A.35}$$

The derivative of the Cauchy strain with respect to the nodal displacements can thus be derived as

$$\begin{aligned}\frac{\partial \epsilon_{ik}}{\partial \mathcal{U}_{jJ}} &= \frac{1}{2}\frac{\partial}{\partial \mathcal{U}_{jJ}}\left(\nabla \mathbf{u} + (\nabla \mathbf{u})^T\right) \\ &= \frac{1}{2}\frac{\partial}{\partial \mathcal{U}_{jJ}}\left(\mathcal{U}_{iI}(\nabla N)_{kI} + \mathcal{U}_{kI}(\nabla N)_{iI}\right) \\ &= \frac{1}{2}\left(\delta_{ij}(\nabla N)_{kJ} + \delta_{kj}(\nabla N)_{iJ}\right). \end{aligned} \tag{A.36}$$

Consequently, the derivation of the Cauchy stress follows as

$$\begin{aligned}\frac{\partial \sigma_{ik}}{\partial \mathcal{U}_{jJ}} &= 2\mu\frac{\partial \epsilon_{ik}}{\partial \mathcal{U}_{jJ}} + \lambda\delta_{ik}\frac{\partial \epsilon_{ll}}{\partial \mathcal{U}_{jJ}} \\ &= \mu\left(\delta_{ij}(\nabla N)_{kJ} + \delta_{kj}(\nabla N)_{iJ}\right) + \frac{\lambda}{2}\delta_{ik}\left(\delta_{lj}(\nabla N)_{lJ} + \delta_{lj}(\nabla N)_{lJ}\right) \\ &= \mu\left(\delta_{ij}(\nabla N)_{kJ} + \delta_{kj}(\nabla N)_{iJ}\right) + \frac{\lambda}{2}2\delta_{ik}(\nabla N)_{jJ} \\ &= \mu\delta_{ij}(\nabla N)_{kJ} + \mu\delta_{kj}(\nabla N)_{iJ} + \lambda\delta_{ik}(\nabla N)_{jJ} \end{aligned} \tag{A.37}$$

and the derivative of the internal force density can be expressed as

$$\begin{aligned}\frac{\partial \hat{f}_{iI}^{X,int}}{\partial \mathcal{U}_{jJ}} &= \frac{\partial}{\partial \mathcal{U}_{jJ}}\left(\sigma_{ik}(\nabla N)_{kI}\right)\mathrm{dV}_0 \\ &= \frac{\partial \sigma_{ik}}{\partial \mathcal{U}_{jJ}}(\nabla N)_{kI} \\ &= \left(\mu\delta_{ij}(\nabla N)_{kJ} + \mu\delta_{kj}(\nabla N)_{iJ} + \lambda\delta_{ik}(\nabla N)_{jJ}\right)(\nabla N_I)_{kI} \\ &= \left(\mu\delta_{ij}(\nabla N)_{kJ} + \mu\delta_{kj}(\nabla N)_{iJ} + \lambda\delta_{ik}(\nabla N)_{jJ}\right)(\nabla N_I)_{kI} \\ &= \mu\delta_{ij}(\nabla N)_{kJ}(\nabla N_I)_{kI} + \mu(\nabla N)_{iJ}(\nabla N_I)_{jI} \\ &\quad +\lambda(\nabla N)_{jJ}(\nabla N_I)_{iI}. \end{aligned} \tag{A.38}$$

This yields the stiffness matrix

$$\frac{\partial f_{iI}^{int}}{\partial \mathcal{U}_{jJ}} = \int_{\Omega_0}\frac{\partial \hat{f}_{iI}^{X,int}}{\partial \mathcal{U}_{jJ}}\mathrm{dV}_0 = \sum_e\int_\tau \frac{\partial \hat{f}_{iI}^{X,int}}{\partial \mathcal{U}_{jJ}}\mathrm{dV}_0 = \sum_e \mathbf{K}^e = \mathbf{K}. \tag{A.39}$$

A.6. Internal nodal forces and the stiffness matrix for corotated elasticity

The polar decomposition of deformation gradient (see section 4.1.3)

$$\mathbf{F} = \mathbf{R}\mathbf{U} \tag{A.40}$$

is used to define the stretch measure

$$\mathbf{U} = \mathbf{R}^T\mathbf{F}. \tag{A.41}$$

We express the displacement gradient through the nodal positions

$$\nabla\mathbf{u} = \mathbf{F} - \mathbf{I} = \nabla(\mathcal{X}_J N_J) = \mathcal{X}_J \nabla N_J - \mathbf{I} \tag{A.42}$$

in order to relate the Cauchy strain to the nodal positions:

$$\begin{aligned}\epsilon &= \frac{1}{2}\left((\mathbf{F}-\mathbf{I}) + (\mathbf{F}-\mathbf{I})^T\right) = \frac{1}{2}\left((\mathcal{X}_J\nabla N_J - \mathbf{I}) + (\mathcal{X}_J\nabla N_J - \mathbf{I})^T\right) \\ &= \frac{1}{2}\left(\mathcal{X}_{iJ}(\nabla N)_{jJ} + \mathcal{X}_{jJ}(\nabla N)_{iJ}\right) - \mathbf{I}.\end{aligned} \tag{A.43}$$

For corotated elasticity, the deformation gradient is replaced by the stretch measure

$$\mathbf{U} = \mathbf{R}^T\nabla\mathbf{F} = R_{ki}\mathcal{X}_{kJ}(\nabla N)_{jJ}. \tag{A.44}$$

Consequently, the corotated Cauchy strain reads

$$\epsilon^{CR} = \epsilon_{ij}^{CR} = \frac{1}{2}\left(\mathbf{R}^T\mathcal{X}_J\nabla N_J + (\mathbf{R}^T\mathcal{X}_J\nabla N_J)^T\right) - \mathbf{I} \tag{A.45}$$

and the corotated stress is derived to

$$\sigma_{ij}^{CR} = 2\mu\epsilon_{ij}^{CR} + \lambda\delta_{ij}\epsilon_{ll}^{CR}.$$

We note that the internal nodal forces can be written in terms of the variation of nodal position

$$\begin{aligned}D_{\delta\mathcal{U}}\Pi(\mathbf{u}_h)_{int} &= \int_{\Omega_0}\sigma : \delta\epsilon \mathrm{dV}_0 = \int_{\Omega_0}\sigma : \frac{1}{2}\left(\delta\nabla\mathbf{u} + (\delta\nabla\mathbf{u})^T\right)\mathrm{dV}_0 \\ &= \int_{\Omega_0}\sigma : \delta\nabla\mathbf{u}\mathrm{dV}_0 = \int_{\Omega_0}\sigma : (\delta\mathcal{U}_I\nabla N_I)\,\mathrm{dV}_0 \\ &= \int_{\Omega_0}\sigma : (\delta\mathcal{X}_I\nabla N_I)\,\mathrm{dV}_0\end{aligned} \tag{A.46}$$

in order to derive the corotated nodal forces

$$\begin{aligned} D_{\delta\mathcal{U}}\Pi(\mathbf{u}_h)_{int} &= \int_{\Omega_0} \sigma : \left(\mathbf{R}^T\delta\mathcal{X}_I\nabla N_I\right)\mathrm{dV}_0 = \int_{\Omega_0} (\mathbf{R}\sigma) : (\delta\mathcal{X}_I\nabla N_I)\,\mathrm{dV}_0 \\ &= \delta\mathcal{X}_{iI}\int_{\Omega_0} \mathbf{R}_{im}\sigma_{mk}(\nabla N)_{kI}\mathrm{dV}_0 = \delta\mathcal{X}_{iI}\int_{\Omega_0} \hat{f}_{iI}^{int,CR}\mathrm{dV}_0 \\ &= \delta\mathcal{X}_{iI}f_{iI}^{int,CR} = \delta\mathcal{X}_I\mathbf{f}_I^{int,CR} \end{aligned} \tag{A.47}$$

with

$$\hat{f}_{iI}^{int,CR} = \int_{\Omega_0} \mathbf{R}_{im}\sigma_{mk}^{CR}(\nabla N)_{kI}\mathrm{dV}_0. \tag{A.48}$$

In order to formulate the corotated stiffness matrix, we first compute the derivate of the corotated Cauchy strain with respect to the nodal positions:

$$\begin{aligned} \frac{\partial\epsilon_{mk}}{\partial\mathcal{X}_{jJ}} &= \frac{1}{2}\frac{\partial}{\partial\mathcal{X}_{jJ}}\left(R_{nm}F_{nk} + F_{nm}R_{nk}\right) - \mathbf{I} \\ &= \frac{1}{2}\frac{\partial}{\partial\mathcal{X}_{jJ}}\left(R_{nm}\mathcal{X}_{nI}\left(\nabla N\right)_{kI} + \mathcal{X}_{nI}\left(\nabla N\right)_{mI}R_{nk}\right) \\ &= \frac{1}{2}\left(\delta_{nj}R_{nm}\left(\nabla N\right)_{kJ} + \delta_{nj}\left(\nabla N\right)_{mJ}R_{nk}\right) \end{aligned} \tag{A.49}$$

In a similar fashion as in the linear elastic case we derive

$$\begin{aligned} &\frac{\partial\sigma_{mk}^{CR}}{\partial\mathcal{X}_{jJ}} = 2\mu\frac{\partial\epsilon_{mk}^{CR}}{\partial\mathcal{X}_{jJ}} + \lambda\delta_{mk}\frac{\partial\epsilon_{ll}^{CR}}{\partial\mathcal{X}_{jJ}} \\ &= \mu\left(\delta_{nj}R_{nm}\left(\nabla N\right)_{kJ} + \delta_{nj}\left(\nabla N\right)_{mJ}R_{nk}\right) \\ &+ \frac{\lambda}{2}\delta_{mk}\left(\delta_{nj}R_{nl}\left(\nabla N\right)_{lJ} + \delta_{nj}\left(\nabla N\right)_{lJ}R_{nl}\right) \\ &= \mu\left(\delta_{nj}R_{nm}\left(\nabla N\right)_{kJ} + \delta_{nj}\left(\nabla N\right)_{mJ}R_{nk}\right) + \lambda\delta_{mk}\delta_{nj}R_{nl}\left(\nabla N\right)_{lJ} \end{aligned} \tag{A.50}$$

and express the corotated force density through

$$
\begin{aligned}
\frac{\partial \hat{f}_{iI}^{X,int}}{\partial \mathcal{X}_{jJ}} &= \frac{\partial}{\partial \mathcal{X}_{jJ}} \mathbf{R}_{im} \sigma_{mk}^{CR} (\nabla N)_{kI} = \mathbf{R}_{im} \frac{\partial \sigma_{mk}^{CR}}{\partial \mathcal{X}_{jJ}} (\nabla N)_{kI} \\
&= \mathbf{R}_{im} \mu \left(\delta_{nj} R_{nm} (\nabla N)_{kJ} + \delta_{nj} (\nabla N)_{mJ} R_{nk} \right) (\nabla N)_{kI} \\
&\quad + \mathbf{R}_{im} \left(\lambda \delta_{mk} \delta_{nj} R_{nl} (\nabla N)_{lJ} \right) (\nabla N)_{kI} \\
&= \mathbf{R}_{im} \mu \left(\delta_{nm} R_{jn} (\nabla N)_{kJ} (\nabla N)_{kI} + (\nabla N)_{mJ} R_{jk} (\nabla N)_{kI} \right) \\
&\quad + \lambda R_{jl} (\nabla N)_{lJ} (\nabla N)_{mI} \\
&= \mathbf{R}_{im} \mu \left(\delta_{nm} (\nabla N)_{kJ} (\nabla N)_{kI} R_{jn} + (\nabla N)_{mJ} (\nabla N)_{nI} \right) R_{jn} \\
&\quad + \lambda (\nabla N)_{nJ} (\nabla N)_{mI} R_{jn} \\
&= \mathbf{R}_{im} \mu \left(\delta_{nm} (\nabla N)_{kJ} (\nabla N)_{kI} + (\nabla N)_{mJ} (\nabla N)_{nI} \right) R_{jn} \\
&\quad + \mathbf{R}_{im} \left(\lambda (\nabla N)_{nJ} (\nabla N)_{mI} \right) R_{jn} \\
&= \mathbf{R}_{im} \frac{\partial \hat{f}_{mI}^{int}}{\partial \mathcal{X}_{nJ}} R_{jn} = \mathbf{R} \frac{\partial \mathbf{f}_I^{int,CR}}{\partial \mathcal{X}_J} \mathbf{R}^T.
\end{aligned}
\tag{A.51}
$$

The global corotated stiffness matrix is then given by

$$
\mathbf{K}^{CR} = \sum_e \int_\tau \frac{\partial \hat{f}_{iI}^{X,int}}{\partial \mathcal{X}_{jJ}} \mathrm{dV}_0 = \sum_e \int_\tau \mathbf{R} \frac{\partial \hat{\mathbf{f}}_I^{int}}{\partial \mathcal{X}_J} \mathbf{R}^T \mathrm{dV}_0. \tag{A.52}
$$

B.

Glossary

$\mathbf{A}$	arbitrary matrix (e.g. system matrix for linear system)
$\mathcal{A}$	additional DOF for sign enriched elements
$\mathcal{B}$	body (object) under analysis
$\mathbf{C}$	Cauchy-Green strain tensor
$\overline{\mathbf{C}}$	modified (isochoric) Cauchy-Green strain tensor
$\mathbf{D}$	damping matrix
$\mathbf{d}$	rate of deformation tensor
$\mathrm{d}\mathbf{A}, \mathrm{dA}\mathbf{n}$	infinitesimal area element in current configuration
$\mathrm{d}\mathbf{A}_0, \mathrm{dA}_0\mathbf{N}$	infinitesimal area element in reference configuration
div	divergence operator in current configuration
Div	divergence operator in reference configuration
dV	infinitesimal volume element in current configuration
dV_0	infinitesimal volume element in reference configuration
$\mathrm{d}\mathbf{x}, \mathrm{d}x_i$	line element in current configuration
$\mathrm{d}\mathbf{X}, \mathrm{d}X_i$	line element in reference configuration
$\mathrm{d}\mathcal{U}$	difference vector of nodal displacements
$\mathrm{d}\dot{\mathcal{U}}$	difference vector of nodal velocities
$\mathrm{d}\chi$	difference vector of nodal positions

Δt	increment during time integration
$\mathbf{E}$	Green-Lagrange strain tensor
$\mathcal{E}$	set of elements in $\mathcal{M}$
ϵ	infinitesimal strain tensor
$\mathbf{f}^{ext}$, $\mathbf{f}_I^{ext}$, f_{iI}^{ext}	vector of external nodal forces
$\mathbf{f}^{int}$, $\mathbf{f}_I^{int}$, f_{iI}^{int}	vector of internal nodal forces
$\hat{f}_{iI}^{X,int}$	internal force density
$\mathbf{f}^{int,CR}$, $\mathbf{f}_I^{int,CR}$, $f_{iI}^{int,CR}$	vector of corotated internal nodal forces
$\hat{f}_{iI}^{int,CR}$	internal force density
$\mathbf{F}$	deformation gradient tensor
$\dot{\mathbf{F}}$	time derivative of the deformation gradient tensor
$\overline{\mathbf{F}}$	modified (isochoric) deformation gradient tensor
Γ_C	boundary of the cut with zero Neumann (force) boundary conditions
Γ_N	boundary with Dirichlet (displacement) boundary conditions
Γ_D	boundary with Neumann (force) boundary conditions
$\mathcal{G}$	Cauchy-elastic response function
grad	gradient operator in current configuration
Grad	gradient operator in reference configuration
$\mathbf{g}$	gravity acceleration vector
$\mathcal{H}$	hyperelastic response function
H	Hamiltonian
$\mathbf{I}$	identity matrix
$\mathbf{l}$	spatial velocity gradient
$\mathbf{K}$	stiffness matrix
$\mathcal{K}$	kinetic energy

L	Lagrangian
$\mathbf{M}$	mass matrix
$\mathcal{M}$	finite element mesh
N_J, N_{jJ}	basis functions
N_I, N_{iI}	test functions
$\mathbf{n}$	normal in current configuration
$\mathbf{N}$	normal in reference configuration
ν	vertex in $\mathcal{S}$
$\mathbf{O}$	lifting operator
Ω_0	region that is occupied by $\mathcal{B}$ in reference configuration
Ω	region that is occupied by $\mathcal{B}$ in current configuration
$\mathbf{P}$	first Piola-Kirchhoff stress tensor
$\mathbf{p}$	point in $\mathcal{B}$
$\mathcal{P}_{ext}$	rate of external mechancial work (power input)
Π	potential energy functional
$\mathcal{P}_{int}$	rate of internal mechanical work
Ψ	internal elastic energy
$\mathbf{R}$	rotation matrix obtained from polar decomposition of $\mathbf{F}$
ρ	densitiy in current configuration
ρ_0	density in reference configuration
$\mathbf{S}$	second Piola-Kirchhoff stress tensor
$\mathcal{S}$	triangular surface mesh
σ	Cauchy stress tensor
$\mathbf{t}$	traction vector in current configuration
$\mathbf{T}$	traction vector in reference configuration
$\mathbb{T}$	element in $\mathcal{S}$
τ	element in $\mathcal{M}$

tr	trace operator
$\mathbf{U}$	stretch matrix obtained from polar decomposition of $\mathbf{F}$
$\mathbf{u}, u_i$	displacement field
$\mathcal{U}, \mathcal{U}_J, \mathcal{U}jJ$	nodal displacement field
$\dot{\mathcal{U}}$	vector of nodal velocities
$\ddot{\mathcal{U}}$	vector of nodal accelerations
$\delta\mathbf{u}$	variation of the displacement field
$\mathbf{w}$	rate of rotation tensor
$\mathbf{v}$	velocity field
$\dot{\mathbf{v}}$	acceleration field
$\mathcal{V}$	set of vertices in $\mathcal{M}$
$V_D(\Gamma_D, \overline{\mathbf{u}})$	space of functions that fulfill the Dirichlet boundary conditions on Γ_D
$V_N(\Gamma_N, \bar{\mathbf{t}})$	space of functions that fulfill the Neumann boundary conditions on Γ_N
w_{int}	stress power per unit reference volume
$\mathbf{x}, x_i$	positional field in the current configuration
$\mathbf{X}, X_i$	positional field in the reference configuration
$\mathcal{X}, \mathcal{X}_J, \mathcal{X}jJ$	nodal positions

List of Figures

List of Tables

Bibliography

[3Di13] 3Dircadb. 3d image reconstruction for comparison of algorithm database. http://www.ircad.fr/softwares/3Dircadb/3Dircadb.php, June 2013.

[ABCM02] Douglas N Arnold, Franco Brezzi, Bernardo Cockburn, and L Donatella Marini. Unified analysis of discontinuous galerkin methods for elliptic problems. *SIAM journal on numerical analysis*, 39(5):1749–1779, 2002.

[ACF11] Jérémie Allard, Hadrien Courtecuisse, and François Faure. Implicit FEM Solver on GPU for Interactive Deformation Simulation. In Wen mei W. Hwu, editor, *GPU Computing Gems Jade Edition*, pages 281–294. Elsevier, November 2011.

[ACW+07] Neculai Archip, Olivier Clatz, Stephen Whalen, Dan Kacher, Andriy Fedorov, Andriy Kot, Nikos Chrisochoides, Ferenc Jolesz, Alexandra Golby, Peter M Black, et al. Non-rigid alignment of pre-operative mri, fmri, and dt-mri with intra-operative mri for enhanced visualization and navigation in image-guided neurosurgery. *Neuroimage*, 35(2):609–624, 2007.

[AGP+06] R. Alterovitz, K. Goldberg, J. Pouliot, I.C.J. Hsu, Y. Kim, S.M. Noworolski, and J. Kurhanewicz. Registration of MR prostate images with biomechanical modeling and nonlinear parameter estimation. *Medical Physics*, 33:446, 2006.

[BC99] Chi-wang Shu Bernardo Cockburn, George E. Karniadakis. The development of discontinuous galerkin methods, 1999.

[BCG+00] J Belgihiti, PA Clavien, E Gadzijev, JO Garden, W Lau, M Makuuchi, et al. The brisbane 2000 terminology of liver anatomy and resections. *Hpb*, 2(3):333–339, 2000.

[BE09] Peter Bastian and Christian Engwer. An unfitted finite element method using discontinuous galerkin. *International journal for numerical methods in engineering*, 79(12):1557–1576, 2009.

[BEK+00] D. Box, D. Ehnebuske, G. Kakivaya, A. Layman, N. Mendelsohn, H.F. Nielsen, S. Thatte, and D. Winer. Simple object access protocol (soap) 1.1. http://www.w3.org/TR/SOAP/, May 2000.

[BFMR08] Matthias Baumhauer, Marco Feuerstein, Hans-Peter Meinzer, and J Rassweiler. Navigation in endoscopic soft tissue surgery: perspectives and limitations. *Journal of Endourology*, 22(4):751–766, 2008.

[BGTG04] Daniel Bielser, Pascal Glardon, Matthias Teschner, and Markus Gross. A state machine for real-time cutting of tetrahedral meshes. *Graphical Models*, 66(6):398–417, 2004.

[BJ05] J. Barbič and D.L. James. Real-time subspace integration for St. Venant-Kirchhoff deformable models. *ACM Transactions on Graphics (TOG)*, 24(3):990, 2005.

[BLM00] T. Belytschko, WK Liu, and B. Moran. *Nonlinear finite elements for continua and structures*, volume 36. Wiley, 2000.

[Bon97] Javier Bonet. *Nonlinear continuum mechanics for finite element analysis*. Cambridge university press, 1997.

[BPH11] Evgeniya Bogatyrenko, Pascal Pompey, and Uwe D Hanebeck. Efficient physics-based tracking of heart surface motion for beating heart surgery robotic systems. *International journal of computer assisted radiology and surgery*, 6(3):387–399, 2011.

[BR97] Francesco Bassi and Stefano Rebay. A high-order accurate discontinuous finite element method for the numerical solution of the compressible navier–stokes equations. *Journal of computational physics*, 131(2):267–279, 1997.

[Bra07] Dietrich Braess. *Finite elements: Theory, fast solvers, and applications in solid mechanics*. Cambridge University Press, 2007.

[BSD+05] KK Brock, MB Sharpe, LA Dawson, SM Kim, and DA Jaffray. Accuracy of finite element model-based multi-organ deformable image registration. *Medical physics*, 32:1647, 2005.

[BTPE06] James Bacon, Neil Tardella, Janey Pratt, and John HUaand James ENGLISH. The surgical simulation and training based language for medical simulation. *Medicine Meets Virtual Reality 14: Accelerating Change in Health Care: Next Medical Toolkit*, 119:37, 2006.

[BW98] D. Baraff and A. Witkin. Large steps in cloth simulation. In *Proceedings of the 25th annual conference on Computer graphics and interactive techniques*, pages 43–54. ACM, 1998.

[CAD+10] H. Courtecuisse, J. Allard, C. Duriez, S. Cotin, et al. Asynchronous preconditioners for efficient solving of non-linear deformations. In *VRIPHYS-Virtual Reality Interaction and Physical Simulation*, pages 59–68, 2010.

[CB97] Rikk Carey and Gavin Bell. *The annotated VRML 2.0 reference manual*. Addison-Wesley Longman Ltd., 1997.

[CBLC02] Mark A Clifford, Filip Banovac, Elliot Levy, and Kevin Cleary. Assessment of hepatic motion secondary to respiration for computer assisted interventions. *Computer Aided Surgery*, 7(5):291–299, 2002.

[CCC+08] Paolo Cignoni, Marco Callieri, Massimiliano Corsini, Matteo Dellepiane, Fabio Ganovelli, and Guido Ranzuglia.

Meshlab: an open-source mesh processing tool. In *Eurographics Italian Chapter Conference*, pages 129–136. The Eurographics Association, 2008.

[CCD+08] Logan W Clements, William C Chapman, Benoit M Dawant, Robert L Galloway Jr, and Michael I Miga. Robust surface registration using salient anatomical features for image-guided liver surgery: Algorithm and validation. *Medical Physics*, 35:2528, 2008.

[CDA00] S. Cotin, H. Delingette, and N. Ayache. A hybrid elastic model for real-time cutting, deformations, and force feedback for surgery training and simulation. *The Visual Computer*, 16(8):437–452, 2000.

[CDC+07] Logan W. Clements, Prashanth Dumpuri, William C. Chapman, Robert L. Galloway, and Michael I. Miga. Atlas-based method for model updating in image-guided liver surgery. In Kevin R. Cleary and Michael I. Miga, editors, *Medical Imaging 2007: Visualization and Image-Guided Procedures*, volume 6509, pages 650917+. SPIE, 2007.

[CDT+05] O. Clatz, H. Delingette, I.F. Talos, AJ Golby, R. Kikinis, FA Jolesz, N. Ayache, SK Warfield, and F. INRIA. Robust nonrigid registration to capture brain shift from intraoperative MRI. *IEEE Transactions on medical imaging*, 24(11):1417–1427, 2005.

[CFK+06] N. Chrisochoides, A. Fedorov, A. Kot, N. Archip, P. Black, O. Clatz, A. Golby, R. Kikinis, and S.K. Warfield. Toward real-time image guided neurosurgery using distributed and grid computing. In *Proceedings of the 2006 ACM/IEEE conference on Supercomputing*, page 76. ACM, 2006.

[CJA+10] H. Courtecuisse, H. Jung, J. Allard, C. Duriez, D.Y. Lee, and S. Cotin. Gpu-based real-time soft tissue deformation with cutting and haptic feedback. *Progress in biophysics and molecular biology*, 103(2):159–168, 2010.

[CK92] AO Cifuentes and A. Kalbag. A performance study of tetrahedral and hexahedral elements in 3-d finite element structural analysis. *Finite Elements in Analysis and Design*, 12(3):313–318, 1992.

[CMG+07] D.M. Cash, M.I. Miga, S.C. Glasgow, B.M. Dawant, L.W. Clements, Z. Cao, R.L. Galloway, and W.C. Chapman. Concepts and preliminary data toward the realization of image-guided liver surgery. *Journal of Gastrointestinal Surgery*, 11(7):844–859, 2007.

[CMJ11] Timothy R Coles, Dwight Meglan, and Nigel W John. The role of haptics in medical training simulators: a survey of the state of the art. *Haptics, IEEE Transactions on*, 4(1):51–66, 2011.

[CMS+05] D.M. Cash, M.I. Miga, T.K. Sinha, R.L. Galloway, and W.C. Chapman. Compensating for intraoperative soft-tissue deformations using incomplete surface data and finite elements. *IEEE transactions on medical imaging*, 24(11):1479–1491, 2005.

[CP04] Matthieu Chabanas and Emmanuel Promayon. Physical model language: Towards a unified representation for continuous and discrete models. In *Medical Simulation*, pages 256–266. Springer, 2004.

[CP08] S. Cotin and J. Passenger. Efficient nonlinear FEM for soft tissue modelling and its GPU implementation within the open source framework SOFA. In *Biomedical Simulation: 4th International Symposium, Isbms 2008, London, Uk, July 7-8, 2008, Proceedings*, page 28. Springer-Verlag New York Inc, 2008.

[CP10] Kevin Cleary and Terry M Peters. Image-guided interventions: technology review and clinical applications. *Annual review of biomedical engineering*, 12:119–142, 2010.

[CPC+07] JR Crouch, SM Pizer, EL Chaney, YC Hu, GS Mageras, and M. Zaider. Automated finite-element analysis for deformable registration of prostate images. *IEEE Transactions on medical imaging*, 26(10):1379, 2007.

[CR03] H. Chui and A. Rangarajan. A new point matching algorithm for non-rigid registration. *Computer Vision and Image Understanding*, 89(2):114–141, 2003.

[CSLY01] Jen-Hui Chuang, Jin-Fa Sheu, Chien-Chou Lin, and Hui-Kuo Yang. Shape matching and recognition using a physically based object model. *Computers & Graphics*, 25(2):211–222, 2001.

[DCDM10] P. Dumpuri, L.W. Clements, B.M. Dawant, and M.I. Miga. Model-updated image-guided liver surgery: Preliminary results using surface characterization. *Progress in biophysics and molecular biology*, 103(2-3):197–207, 2010.

[DGW11a] C. Dick, J. Georgii, and R. Westermann. A real-time multigrid finite hexahedra method for elasticity simulation using cuda. *Simulation Modelling Practice and Theory*, 19(2):801–816, 2011.

[DGW11b] Christian Dick, Joachim Georgii, and Rüdiger Westermann. A hexahedral multigrid approach for simulating cuts in deformable objects. *Visualization and Computer Graphics, IEEE Transactions on*, 17(11):1663–1675, 2011.

[dSGF+12] Thiago R dos Santos, Caspar J Goch, Alfred M Franz, Hans-Peter Meinzer, Tobias Heimann, and Lena Maier-Hein. Minimally deformed correspondences between surfaces for intra-operative registration. In *Proceedings of SPIE*, volume 8314, page 83141C, 2012.

[dSSK+14] Thiago Ramos dos Santos, Alexander Seitel, Thomas Kilgus, Stefan Suwelack, Anna-Laura Wekerle, Hannes Kenngott, Stefanie Speidel, Heinz-Peter Schlemmer, Hans-Peter Meinzer, Tobias Heimann, et al. Pose-independent surface matching for intra-operative soft-tissue markerless registration. *Medical Image Analysis*, 2014.

[ECL08] A.T. Eyck, F. Celiker, and A. Lew. Adaptive stabilization of discontinuous Galerkin methods for nonlinear elasticity: Motivation, formulation, and numerical examples.

Computer Methods in Applied Mechanics and Engineering, 197(45-48):3605–3622, 2008.

[FB10] Thomas-Peter Fries and Ted Belytschko. The extended/-generalized finite element method: An overview of the method and its applications. *International Journal for Numerical Methods in Engineering*, 84(3):253–304, 2010.

[FDD+12] F. Faure, C. Duriez, H. Delingette, J. Allard, B. Gilles, S. Marchesseau, H. Talbot, H. Courtecuisse, G. Bousquet, I. Peterlik, et al. Sofa: A multi-model framework for interactive physical simulation. *Soft Tissue Biomechanical Modeling for Computer Assisted Surgery*, pages 283–321, 2012.

[FDKP12] Céline Fouard, Aurélien Deram, Yannick Keraval, and Emmanuel Promayon. Camitk: a modular framework integrating visualization, image processing and biomechanical modeling. In *Soft Tissue Biomechanical Modeling for Computer Assisted Surgery*, pages 323–354. Springer, 2012.

[FH05] CA Felippa and B. Haugen. A unified formulation of small-strain corotational finite elements: I. Theory. *Computer methods in applied mechanics and engineering*, 194(21-24):2285–2335, 2005.

[FMHN08] Marco Feuerstein, Thomas Mussack, Sandro Michael Heining, and Nassir Navab. Intraoperative laparoscope augmentation for port placement and resection planning in minimally invasive liver resection. *Medical Imaging, IEEE Transactions on*, 27(3):355–369, 2008.

[FP09] Andreas Fabri and Sylvain Pion. Cgal: The computational geometry algorithms library. In *Proceedings of the 17th ACM SIGSPATIAL international conference on advances in geographic information systems*, pages 538–539. ACM, 2009.

[Fun93] Y.C. Fung. *Biomechanics: mechanical properties of living tissues*. Springer, 1993.

[GAA+12] Alfredo D Guerron, Shamil Aliyev, Orhan Agcaoglu, Erol Aksoy, Halit Eren Taskin, Federico Aucejo, Charles Miller,

John Fung, and Eren Berber. Laparoscopic versus open resection of colorectal liver metastasis. *Surgical endoscopy*, pages 1–6, 2012.

[GLS99] William Gropp, Ewing Lusk, and Anthony Skjellum. *Using MPI: portable parallel programming with the message-passing interface*, volume 1. MIT press, 1999.

[GNK+01] David T Gering, Arya Nabavi, Ron Kikinis, Noby Hata, Lauren J O'Donnell, W Eric L Grimson, Ferenc A Jolesz, Peter M Black, and William M Wells. An integrated visualization system for surgical planning and guidance using image fusion and an open mr. *Journal of Magnetic Resonance Imaging*, 13(6):967–975, 2001.

[GW08] Joachim Georgii and Rüdiger Westermann. Corotated finite elements made fast and stable. In *Proceedings of the 5th Workshop On Virtual Reality Interaction and Physical Simulation*, pages 11–19, 2008.

[GWB08] R. Gracie, H. Wang, and T. Belytschko. Blending in the extended finite element method by discontinuous Galerkin and assumed strain methods. *International Journal for Numerical Methods in Engineering*, 74(11):1645–1669, 2008.

[GWL99] Hartmut K Gumprecht, Darius C Widenka, and Christianto B Lumenta. Brainlab vectorvision neuronavigation system: technology and clinical experiences in 131 cases. *Neurosurgery*, 44(1):97–104, 1999.

[H+94] Thomas JR Hughes et al. *Mathematical foundations of elasticity*. DoverPublications. com, 1994.

[HAL04] Amy Henderson, Jim Ahrens, and Charles Law. *The ParaView Guide*. Kitware Clifton Park, NY, 2004.

[HAT+12] Yipeng Hu, Hashim Uddin Ahmed, Zeike Taylor, Clare Allen, Mark Emberton, David Hawkes, and Dean Barratt. Mr to ultrasound registration for image-guided prostate interventions. *Medical image analysis*, 16(3):687–703, 2012.

[HDB+13] Nazim Haouchine, Jérémie Dequidt, Marie-Odile Berger, Stéphane Cotin, et al. Deformation-based augmented reality for hepatic surgery. In *Medicine Meets Virtual Reality, MMVR 20*, 2013.

[HDP+13] Nazim Haouchine, Jérémie Dequidt, Igor Peterlik, Erwan Kerrien, Marie-Odile Berger, Stéphane Cotin, et al. Image-guided simulation of heterogeneous tissue deformation for augmented reality during hepatic surgery. In *ISMAR-IEEE International Symposium on Mixed and Augmented Reality 2013*, 2013.

[HG01] G.A. Holzapfel and T.C. Gasser. A viscoelastic model for fiber-reinforced composites at finite strains: Continuum basis, computational aspects and applications. *Computer methods in applied mechanics and engineering*, 190(34):4379–4403, 2001.

[HHMM+13] Archie Hughes-Hallett, Erik K Mayer, Hani J Marcus, Thomas P Cundy, Philip J Pratt, Ara W Darzi, and Justin A Vale. Augmented reality partial nephrectomy: Examining the current status and future perspectives. *Urology*, 2013.

[HJST13] Jan Hegemann, Chenfanfu Jiang, Craig Schroeder, and Joseph M Teran. A level set method for ductile fracture. In *Proceedings of the 12th ACM SIGGRAPH/Eurographics Symposium on Computer Animation*, pages 193–201. ACM, 2013.

[HLBT12] Nikolai Hungr, Jean-Alexandre Long, Vincent Beix, and Jocelyne Troccaz. A realistic deformable prostate phantom for multimodal imaging and needle-insertion procedures. *Medical Physics*, 39:2031, 2012.

[HN03] Stefan Hartmann and Patrizio Neff. Polyconvexity of generalized polynomial-type hyperelastic strain energy functions for near-incompressibility. *International Journal of Solids and Structures*, 40(11):2767–2791, 2003.

[HNF+06] A. Hostettler, SA Nicolau, C. Forest, L. Soler, and Y. Remond. Real time simulation of organ motions induced by breathing: First evaluation on patient data. *Lecture Notes in Computer Science*, 4072:9, 2006.

[HNS+08] A. Hostettler, S.A. Nicolau, L. Soler, Y. Rémond, and J. Marescaux. A Real-Time Predictive Simulation of Abdominal Organ Positions Induced by Free Breathing. *Lecture Notes in Computer Science*, 5104:89–97, 2008.

[Hol00] G.A. Holzapfel. *Nonlinear solid mechanics*. Wiley New York, 2000.

[HPE+07] Mingxing Hu, Graeme Penney, Philip Edwards, Michael Figl, and David J Hawkes. 3d reconstruction of internal organ surfaces for minimal invasive surgery. In *Medical Image Computing and Computer-Assisted Intervention–MICCAI 2007*, pages 68–77. Springer, 2007.

[HS88] Nicholas J. Higham and Robert S. Schreiber. Fast polar decomposition of an arbitrary matrix. Technical report, Cornell University, Ithaca, NY, USA, 1988.

[HS04] Michael Hauth and Wolfgang Strasser. Corotational simulation of deformable solids. In *J. Winter School of Computer Graphics*, pages 137–145, 2004.

[Hub11] Maik Huber. Extended fem basierend auf der unstetigen ggalerkin methode zur simulation chirurgischer schnitte in weichgewebe. Master's thesis, Karlsruhe Institute of Technology, 2011.

[HWM06] T. Hawkins, A. Wittek, and K. Miller. Comparison of constitutive models of brain tissue for non-rigid image registration. In *2nd Workshop on Computer Assisted Diagnosis and Surgery*, 2006.

[Ibr09] Adnan Ibrahimbegović. *Nonlinear solid mechanics: theoretical formulations and finite element solution methods*, volume 160. Springer, 2009.

[JBB+10] L. Jerabkova, G. Bousquet, S. Barbier, F. Faure, and J. Allard. Volumetric modeling and interactive cutting of deformable bodies. *Progress in biophysics and molecular biology*, 2010.

[JGMJ06] Pierre Jannin, Christophe Grova, and Calvin R Maurer Jr. Model for defining and reporting reference-based validation protocols in medical image processing. *International Journal of Computer Assisted Radiology and Surgery*, 1(2):63–73, 2006.

[JK09] L. Jerabkova and T. Kuhlen. Stable cutting of deformable objects in virtual environments using XFEM. *Computer Graphics and Applications, IEEE*, 29(2):61–71, 2009.

[JSZH09] P. Jordan, S. Socrate, TE Zickler, and RD Howe. Constitutive modeling of porcine liver in indentation using 3D ultrasound imaging. *Journal of the Mechanical Behavior of Biomedical Materials*, 2(2):192–201, 2009.

[JWM08] Grand Roman Joldes, Adam Wittek, and Karol Miller. Suite of finite element algorithms for accurate computation of soft tissue deformation for surgical simulation, 2008.

[JWR04] Andrei C Jalba, Michael HF Wilkinson, and Jos BTM Roerdink. Cpm: A deformable model for shape recovery and segmentation based on charged particles. *Pattern Analysis and Machine Intelligence, IEEE Transactions on*, 26(10):1320–1335, 2004.

[KCO+03] A.E. Kerdok, S.M. Cotin, M.P. Ottensmeyer, A.M. Galea, R.D. Howe, and S.L. Dawson. Truth cube: Establishing physical standards for soft tissue simulation. *Medical Image Analysis*, 7(3):283–291, 2003.

[KDE+12] Markus Kleemann, Steffen Deichmann, Hamed Esnaashari, Armin Besirevic, Osama Shahin, Hans-Peter Bruch, and Tilman Laubert. Laparoscopic navigated liver resection: Technical aspects and clinical practice in benign liver tumors. *Case reports in surgery*, 2012, 2012.

[KMAB04] Alexander F Kolen, Naomi R Miller, Eltayeb E Ahmed, and Jeffrey C Bamber. Characterization of cardiovascular liver motion for the eventual application of elasticity imaging to the liver in vivo. *Physics in medicine and biology*, 49(18):4187, 2004.

[KMB+09] P. Kaufmann, S. Martin, M. Botsch, E. Grinspun, and M. Gross. Enrichment textures for detailed cutting of shells. *ACM Transactions on Graphics (TOG)*, 28(3):50, 2009.

[KMBG09] P. Kaufmann, S. Martin, M. Botsch, and M. Gross. Flexible simulation of deformable models using discontinuous Galerkin FEM. *Graphical Models*, 2009.

[KRS09] I. Khalaji, K. Rahemifar, and A. Samani. Accelerated statistical shape model-based technique for tissue deformation estimation. In *Proceedings of SPIE*, volume 7261, page 72610U, 2009.

[KS05] J. Kim and M.A. Srinivasan. Characterization of viscoelastic soft tissue properties from in vivo animal experiments and inverse FE parameter estimation. *Medical Image Computing and Computer-Assisted Intervention–MICCAI 2005*, pages 599–606, 2005.

[KVPP10] Mitsuhiro Kawata, Nikolay V Vasilyev, Douglas P Perrin, and J Pedro. Beating-heart mitral valve suture annuloplasty under real-time three-dimensional echocardiography guidance: an ex vivo study. *Interactive cardiovascular and thoracic surgery*, 11(1):6–9, 2010.

[KWG+13a] Darko Katić, Anna-Laura Wekerle, Jochen Görtler, Patrick Spengler, Sebastian Bodenstedt, Sebastian Röhl, Stefan Suwelack, Hannes Götz Kenngott, Martin Wagner, Beat Peter Müller-Stich, et al. Context-aware augmented reality in laparoscopic surgery. *Computerized Medical Imaging and Graphics*, 37(2):174–182, 2013.

[KWG+13b] Hannes G Kenngott, Martin Wagner, Matthias Gondan, Felix Nickel, Marco Nolden, Andreas Fetzer, Jürgen Weitz,

Lars Fischer, Stefanie Speidel, Hans-Peter Meinzer, et al. Real-time image guidance in laparoscopic liver surgery: first clinical experience with a guidance system based on intraoperative ct imaging. *Surgical endoscopy*, pages 1–8, 2013.

[KY93] L.Y. Kolotilina and A.Y. Yeremin. Factorized sparse approximate inverse preconditionings i. theory. *SIAM Journal on Matrix Analysis and Applications*, 14(1):45–58, 1993.

[KYF05] Christian Kanzow, Nobuo Yamashita, and Masao Fukushima. Levenberg–marquardt methods with strong local convergence properties for solving nonlinear equations with convex constraints. *Journal of Computational and Applied Mathematics*, 173(2):321–343, 2005.

[KZHCO10] O.V. Kaick, H. Zhang, G. Hamarneh, and D. Cohen-Or. A survey on shape correspondence. In *Computer Graphics Forum*, volume 20, pages 1–23, 2010.

[LF09] Yaron Lipman and Thomas Funkhouser. Möbius voting for surface correspondence. In *ACM Transactions on Graphics (TOG)*, volume 28, page 72. ACM, 2009.

[LGD10] K. Lister, Z. Gao, and J.P. Desai. Development of In Vivo Constitutive Models for Liver: Application to Surgical Simulation. *Annals of biomedical engineering*, pages 1–14, 2010.

[Lip11] Herbert Lippert. *Lehrbuch Anatomie*. Elsevier, Urban&FischerVerlag, 2011.

[LLCO08] Yaron Lipman, David Levin, and Daniel Cohen-Or. Green coordinates. *ACM Trans. Graph.*, 27(3):78:1–78:10, August 2008.

[LNSO04] A. Lew, P. Neff, D. Sulsky, and M. Ortiz. Optimal BV estimates for a discontinuous Galerkin method for linear elasticity, 2004.

[Lou04] M.I.A. Lourakis. levmar: Levenberg-marquardt nonlinear least squares algorithms in C/C++. [web page] `http://www.ics.forth.gr/~lourakis/levmar/`, Jul. 2004. [Accessed on 31 Jan. 2005.].

[LST09] S.H. Lee, E. Sifakis, and D. Terzopoulos. Comprehensive biomechanical modeling and simulation of the upper body. *ACM Transactions on Graphics (TOG)*, 28(4):99, 2009.

[LVR+12] Thomas Langø, Sinara Vijayan, Anna Rethy, Cecilie Våpenstad, Ole Vegard Solberg, Ronald Mårvik, Gjermund Johnsen, and Toril N Hernes. Navigated laparoscopic ultrasound in abdominal soft tissue surgery: technological overview and perspectives. *International journal of computer assisted radiology and surgery*, 7(4):585–599, 2012.

[MC97] K. Miller and K. Chinzei. Constitutive modelling of brain tissue: experiment and theory. *Journal of Biomechanics*, 30(11-12):1115–1121, 1997.

[MDB99] Nicolas Moës, John Dolbow, and Ted Belytschko. A finite element method for crack growth without remeshing. *International Journal for Numerical Methods in Engineering*, 46(1):131–150, 1999.

[MEAW12] Steve A Maas, Benjamin J Ellis, Gerard A Ateshian, and Jeffrey A Weiss. Febio: finite elements for biomechanics. *Journal of biomechanical engineering*, 134(1), 2012.

[MG04] M. Muller and M. Gross. Interactive virtual materials. In *Proceedings- Graphics Interface*. CANADIAN INFORMATION PROCESSING SOCIETY, 1 Yonge St, 2401, Toronto, ON M 5 E 1 E 5, Canada, 2004.

[MHMB+13] Lena Maier-Hein, Peter Mountney, A Bartoli, H Elhawary, D Elson, Anja Groch, A Kolb, Marcos Rodrigues, J Sorger, Stefanie Speidel, et al. Optical techniques for 3d surface reconstruction in computer-assisted laparoscopic surgery. *Medical image analysis*, 17(8):974–996, 2013.

[Mil00] K. Miller. Constitutive modelling of abdominal organs. *Journal of Biomechanics*, 33(3):367–373, 2000.

[MJLW07] K. Miller, G. Joldes, D. Lance, and A. Wittek. Total Lagrangian explicit dynamics finite element algorithm for computing soft tissue deformation. *Communications in numerical methods in engineering*, 23(2):121–134, 2007.

[MKSN+12] Seyed Reza Mousavi, Iman Khalaji, Ali Sadeghi Naini, Kaamran Raahemifar, and Abbas Samani. Statistical finite element method for real-time tissue mechanics analysis. *Computer methods in biomechanics and biomedical engineering*, 15(6):595–608, 2012.

[MMD+04] Y Munz, K Moorthy, A Dosis, JD Hernandez, S Bann, F Bello, S Martin, A Darzi, and T Rockall. The benfits of stereoscopic vision in robotic-assisted performance on bench models. *Surgical Endoscopy And Other Interventional Techniques*, 18(4):611–616, 2004.

[MS97] A. Mazura and S. Seifert. Virtual cutting in medical data. *Studies in health technology and informatics*, 39:420, 1997.

[MS10] Andriy Myronenko and Xubo Song. Point set registration: Coherent point drift. *Pattern Analysis and Machine Intelligence, IEEE Transactions on*, 32(12):2262–2275, 2010.

[MTPS09] J. Mezger, B. Thomaszewski, S. Pabst, and W. Straßer. Interactive physically-based shape editing. *Computer Aided Geometric Design*, 26(6):680–694, 2009.

[MY12] Peter Mountney and Guang-Zhong Yang. Context specific descriptors for tracking deforming tissue. *Medical Image Analysis*, 16(3):550–561, 2012.

[NACC08] S. Niroomandi, I. Alfaro, E. Cueto, and F. Chinesta. On the Application of Model Reduction Techniques to Real-Time Simulation of Non-linear tissues. *Lecture Notes in Computer Science*, 5104:11–18, 2008.

[NGG09] Kevin Tri Nguyen, T Clark Gamblin, and David A Geller. World review of laparoscopic liver resection-2,804 patients. *Annals of surgery*, 250(5):831–841, 2009.

[NHS+07] Masahiko Nakamoto, Hiroaki Hirayama, Yoshinobu Sato, Kozo Konishi, Yoshihiro Kakeji, Makoto Hashizume, and Shinichi Tamura. Recovery of respiratory motion and deformation of the liver using laparoscopic freehand 3d ultrasound system. *Medical image analysis*, 11(5):429–442, 2007.

[NKJF09] Matthieu Nesme, Paul G Kry, Lenka Jeřábková, and François Faure. Preserving topology and elasticity for embedded deformable models. In *ACM Transactions on Graphics (TOG)*, volume 28, page 52. ACM, 2009.

[NME+09] David P Noonan, Peter Mountney, Daniel S Elson, Ara Darzi, and Guang-Zhong Yang. A stereoscopic fibroscope for camera motion and 3d depth recovery during minimally invasive surgery. In *Robotics and Automation, 2009. ICRA'09. IEEE International Conference on*, pages 4463–4468. IEEE, 2009.

[NMHB04] A. Nava, E. Mazza, O. Haefner, and M. Bajka. Experimental observation and modelling of preconditioning in soft biological tissues. *Lecture Notes in Computer Science*, 3078:1–8, 2004.

[NNZ+10] Kazuhiro Nakamura, Yukio Naya, Satoki Zenbutsu, Kazuhiro Araki, Shuko Cho, Sho Ohta, Naoki Nihei, Hiroyoshi Suzuki, Tomohiko Ichikawa, and Tatsuo Igarashi. Surgical navigation using three-dimensional computed tomography images fused intraoperatively with live video*. *Journal of Endourology*, 24(4):521–524, 2010.

[NSMM11] Stéphane Nicolau, Luc Soler, Didier Mutter, and Jacques Marescaux. Augmented reality in laparoscopic surgical oncology. *Surgical oncology*, 20(3):189–201, 2011.

[NW99] Jorge Nocedal and Stephen J Wright. *Numerical optimization*. Springer verlag, 1999.

[Ogd97] Raymond W Ogden. *Non-linear elastic deformations*. Courier Dover Publications, 1997.

[PC08] Terry Peters and Kevin Cleary. *Image-guided interventions: technology and applications*. Springer, 2008.

[Per07] Philippe L Pereira. Actual role of radiofrequency ablation of liver metastases. *European radiology*, 17(8):2062–2070, 2007.

[PFtH+08] Kirsten M Pondman, Jurgen J Fütterer, Bennie ten Haken, Leo J Schultze Kool, J Alfred Witjes, Thomas Hambrock, Katarzyna J Macura, and Jelle O Barentsz. Mr-guided biopsy of the prostate: an overview of techniques and a systematic review. *European urology*, 54(3):517–527, 2008.

[PHK04] Steve Pieper, Michael Halle, and Ron Kikinis. 3d slicer. In *Biomedical Imaging: Nano to Macro, 2004. IEEE International Symposium on*, pages 632–635. IEEE, 2004.

[PMV+12] Philip Pratt, Erik Mayer, Justin Vale, Daniel Cohen, Eddie Edwards, Ara Darzi, and Guang-Zhong Yang. An effective visualisation and registration system for image-guided robotic partial nephrectomy. *Journal of Robotic Surgery*, 6(1):23–31, 2012.

[PSDH10] B. Pfau, S. Suwelack, R. Dillmann, and V. Heuveline. Soft tissue simulation using discontinuous galerkin fem. In *RICAM Workshop on Discontinuous Galerkin Methods*, 2010.

[PSS+14] C. Paulus, S. Suwelack, N. Schoch, S. Speidel, and V. Dillmann, R.and Heuveline. Simulation of arbitrary cuts in soft tissue with the extended finite element method (xfem). *Preprint Series of the Engineering Mathematics and Computing Lab)*, 2014.

[PSVSY10] P. Pratt, D. Stoyanov, M. Visentini-Scarzanella, and G.Z. Yang. Dynamic Guidance for Robotic Surgery Using Image-Constrained Biomechanical Models. *Medical Image Computing and Computer-Assisted Intervention–MICCAI 2010*, pages 77–85, 2010.

[RBK+12] S. Röhl, S. Bodenstedt, C. Küderle, S. Suwelack, H. Kenngott, BP Müller-Stich, R. Dillmann, and S. Speidel. Fusion of intraoperative force sensoring, surface reconstruction and biomechanical modeling. In *Proc. SPIE Medical Imaging*, 2012.

[RBS+12] Sebastian Röhl, Sebastian Bodenstedt, Stefan Suwelack, Hannes Kenngott, Beat P Müller-Stich, Rüdiger Dillmann, and Stefanie Speidel. Dense gpu-enhanced surface reconstruction from stereo endoscopic images for intraoperative registration. *Medical Physics*, 39:1632, 2012.

[RES10] S. Raghunathan, D. Evans, and J.L. Sparks. Poroviscoelastic Modeling of Liver Biomechanical Response in Unconfined Compression. *Annals of biomedical engineering*, 38(5):1789–1800, 2010.

[RL01] S. Rusinkiewicz and M. Levoy. Efficient variants of the icp algorithm. In *3-D Digital Imaging and Modeling, 2001. Proceedings. Third International Conference on*, pages 145–152. IEEE, 2001.

[RLB09] R. Rangarajan, A. Lew, and G.C. Buscaglia. A discontinuous-galerkin-based immersed boundary method with non-homogeneous boundary conditions and its application to elasticity. *Computer Methods in Applied Mechanics and Engineering*, 198(17-20):1513–1534, 2009.

[RMOZ04] Torsten Rohlfing, Calvin Maurer, Walter O'Dell, and Jianhui Zhong. Modeling liver motion and deformation during the respiratory cycle using intensity-based nonrigid registration of gated mr images. *Medical physics*, 31:427, 2004.

[RPL08] Rogério Richa, Philippe Poignet, and Chao Liu. Deformable motion tracking of the heart surface. In *Intelligent Robots and Systems, 2008. IROS 2008. IEEE/RSJ International Conference on*, pages 3997–4003. IEEE, 2008.

[RRA12] Ahsan Rao, Ghaus Rao, and Irfan Ahmed. Laparoscopic vs. open liver resection for malignant liver disease. a systematic review. *The Surgeon*, 10(4):194–201, 2012.

[RWC$^+$13] D Rucker, Y Wu, L Clements, J Ondrake, T Pheiffer, A Simpson, W Jarnagin, and M Miga. A mechanics-based nonrigid registration method for liver surgery using sparse intraoperative data. *IEEE transactions on medical imaging*, 2013.

[SAFP04] KJM Surry, HJB Austin, A Fenster, and TM Peters. Poly (vinyl alcohol) cryogel phantoms for use in ultrasound and mr imaging. *Physics in medicine and biology*, 49(24):5529, 2004.

[SB00] Natarajan Sukumar and Ted Belytschko. Arbitrary branched and intersecting cracks with the extended finite element method. *Int. J. Numer. Meth. Engng*, 48:1741–1760, 2000.

[SBKK12] Pirmin Storz, Gerhard F Buess, Wolfgang Kunert, and Andreas Kirschniak. 3d hd versus 2d hd: surgical task efficiency in standardised phantom tasks. *Surgical endoscopy*, 26(5):1454–1460, 2012.

[SBKS14] Osama Shahin, Armin Beširević, Markus Kleemann, and Alexander Schlaefer. Ultrasound-based tumor movement compensation during navigated laparoscopic liver interventions. *Surgical endoscopy*, pages 1–8, 2014.

[SBvDS12] Rutger M Schols, Nicole D Bouvy, Ronald M van Dam, and Laurents PS Stassen. Advanced intraoperative imaging methods for laparoscopic anatomy navigation: an overview. *Surgical endoscopy*, pages 1–9, 2012.

[SDF07] Eftychios Sifakis, Kevin G Der, and Ronald Fedkiw. Arbitrary cutting of deformable tetrahedralized objects. In *Proceedings of the 2007 ACM SIGGRAPH/Eurographics symposium on Computer animation*, pages 73–80. Eurographics Association, 2007.

[SDJM12] Amber L Simpson, Prashanth Dumpuri, William R Jarnagin, and Michael I Miga. Model-assisted image-guided liver surgery using sparse intraoperative data. In *Soft Tissue Biomechanical Modeling for Computer Assisted Surgery*, pages 7–40. Springer, 2012.

[SHHM$^+$13] Ashwin N Sridhar, Archie Hughes-Hallett, Erik K Mayer, Philip J Pratt, Philip J Edwards, Guang-Zhong Yang, Ara W Darzi, and Justin A Vale. Image-guided robotic interventions for prostate cancer. *Nature Reviews Urology*, 2013.

[SK04] Alla Sheffer and Vladislav Kraevoy. Pyramid coordinates for morphing and deformation. In *3D Data Processing, Visualization and Transmission, 2004. 3DPVT 2004. Proceedings. 2nd International Symposium on*, pages 68–75. IEEE, 2004.

[SKW$^+$12] S. Suwelack, D. Katic, S. Wagner, P. Spengler, S. Bodenstedt, S. Röhl, R. Dillmann, and S. Speidel. Lightweight distributed computing for intraoperative real-time image guidance. In *Proc. SPIE Medical Imaging*, 2012.

[SKX$^+$08] Anurag K Singh, Jochen Kruecker, Sheng Xu, Neil Glossop, Peter Guion, Karen Ullman, Peter L Choyke, and Bradford J Wood. Initial clinical experience with real-time transrectal ultrasonography-magnetic resonance imaging fusion-guided prostate biopsy. *BJU international*, 101(7):841–845, 2008.

[SLH$^+$13] S. Suwelack, D. Lukarski, V. Heuveline, R. Dillmann, and S. Speidel. Accurate surface embedding for higher order finite elements. In *Symposium on Computer Animation*, 2013.

[SM03] Endre Süli and David F Mayers. *An introduction to numerical analysis*. Cambridge University Press, 2003.

[SRB$^+$13] S. Suwelack, S. Röhl, S. Bodenstedt, D. Katic, H. Kenngott, B. Mueller-Stich, A. Wekerle, M. Wagner, J. Wünscher, R. Dillmann, L. Maier-Hein, and S. Speidel. Biomechanical simulations, soft tissue phantoms and open data - validating and benchmarking systems for computer assisted minimally invasive surgery. In *CRAS*, 2013.

[SRB+14] Stefan Suwelack, Sebastian Röhl, Sebastian Bodenstedt, Daniel Reichard, Rüdiger Dillmann, Thiago dos Santos, Lena Maier-Hein, Martin Wagner, Josephine Wünscher, Hannes Kenngott, et al. Physics-based shape matching for intraoperative image guidance. *Medical physics*, 41(11):111901, 2014.

[SRD+11] S. Suwelack, S. Roehl, R. Dillmann, A. Wekerle, H. Kenngott, B. Müller-Stich, C. Alt, and S. Speidel. Quadratic corotated finite elements for real-time soft tissue registration. In *MICCAI workshop: Computational Biomechanics for Medicine*. Springer, 2011.

[SS02] Daniel Scharstein and Richard Szeliski. Middlebury stereo vision page. *Online at http://www. middlebury. edu/stereo*, 2002.

[SSDH13] N. Schoch, S. Suwelack, R. Dillmann, and V. Heuveline. Simulation of surgical cutting of soft tissue using the x-fem. *Preprint Series of the Engineering Mathematics and Computing Lab*, 2013.

[SSND01] O.M. Skrinjar, C. Studholme, A. Nabavi, and J.S. Duncan. Steps Toward a Stereo-Camera-Guided Biomechanical Model for Brain Shift Compensation. In *Proceedings of the 17th International Conference on Information Processing in Medical Imaging*, pages 183–189. Springer-Verlag London, UK, 2001.

[SSPY10] Danail Stoyanov, Marco Visentini Scarzanella, Philip Pratt, and Guang-Zhong Yang. Real-time stereo reconstruction in robotically assisted minimally invasive surgery. In *Proceedings of the 13th international conference on Medical image computing and computer-assisted intervention: Part I*, pages 275–282. Springer-Verlag, 2010.

[SSRD10] S. Suwelack, S. Speidel, S. Roehl, and R. Dillmann. Towards finite element-based soft tissue modelling for real-time image registration. In *Proc. Computer Assisted Radiology and Surgery (CARS)*, 2010.

[SSS+14] S. Suwelack, C. Sander, J. Schill, M. Serf, M. Danz, T. Asfour, W. Burger, R. Dillmann, and S. Speidel. Towards open source, low-cost haptics for surgery simulation. In *Medicine Meets Virtual Reality*, 2014.

[Sto12] Danail Stoyanov. Surgical vision. *Annals of biomedical engineering*, pages 1–14, 2012.

[STR+11] S. Suwelack, H. Talbot, S. Röhl, R. Dillmann, and S. Speidel. A biomechanical liver model for intraoperative soft tissue registration. In *Proc. SPIE Medical Imaging*, 2011.

[SY07] Danail Stoyanov and Guang-Zhong Yang. Stabilization of image motion for robotic assisted beating heart surgery. In *Medical Image Computing and Computer-Assisted Intervention 2007*, pages 417–424. Springer, 2007.

[TCC+08] ZA Taylor, O. Comas, M. Cheng, J. Passenger, DJ Hawkes, D. Atkinson, and S. Ourselin. On modelling of anisotropic viscoelasticity for soft tissue simulation: Numerical solution and GPU execution. *Medical Image Analysis*, 2008.

[TCL+13] Gary KL Tam, Zhi-Quan Cheng, Yu-Kun Lai, Frank C Langbein, Yonghuai Liu, David Marshall, Ralph R Martin, Xian-Fang Sun, and Paul L Rosin. Registration of 3d point clouds and meshes: A survey from rigid to nonrigid. *Visualization and Computer Graphics, IEEE Transactions on*, 19(7):1199–1217, 2013.

[TCO08] ZA Taylor, M. Cheng, and S. Ourselin. High-speed nonlinear finite element analysis for surgical simulation using graphics processing units. *IEEE Transactions on Medical Imaging*, 27(5):650–663, 2008.

[TEL06] A. Ten Eyck and A. Lew. *Discontinuous Galerkin methods for non-linear elasticity*, volume 67. John Wiley & Sons, Ltd. Chichester, UK, 2006.

[TFD+10] J. Tokuda, G.S. Fischer, S.P. DiMaio, D.G. Gobbi, C. Csoma, P.W. Mewes, G. Fichtinger, C.M. Tempany, and N. Hata. Integrated navigation and control software system for mri-guided robotic prostate interventions. *Computerized Medical Imaging and Graphics*, 34(1):3–8, 2010.

[TFP+09] J. Tokuda, G.S. Fischer, X. Papademetris, Z. Yaniv, L. Ibanez, P. Cheng, H. Liu, J. Blevins, J. Arata, A.J. Golby, et al. Openigtlink: an open network protocol for image-guided therapy environment. *The International Journal of Medical Robotics and Computer Assisted Surgery*, 5(4):423–434, 2009.

[TMY+11] Min Tang, Dinesh Manocha, Sung-Eui Yoon, Peng Du, Jae-Pil Heo, and Ruo-Feng Tong. Volccd: Fast continuous collision culling between deforming volume meshes. *ACM Transactions on Graphics (TOG)*, 30(5):111, 2011.

[TSF+07] Nicolas Toussaint, Jean-Christophe Souplet, Pierre Fillard, et al. Medinria: Medical image navigation and research tool by inria. In *Proc. of MICCAI*, volume 7, 2007.

[Vig09] Lara M. Vigneron. *FEM/XFEM-Based Modeling of Brain Shift, Resection, and Retraction for Image-Guided Surgery*. PhD thesis, University of Liège,, 2009.

[Vin97] S. Vinoski. Corba: Integrating diverse applications within distributed heterogeneous environments. *Communications Magazine, IEEE*, 35(2):46–55, 1997.

[VWRV11] L.M. Vigneron, S.K. Warfield, P.A. Robe, and J.G. Verly. 3D XFEM-based modeling of retraction for preoperative image update. *Computer Aided Surgery*, 16(3):121–134, 2011.

[WBS+12] Daniel Weber, Jan Bender, Markus Schnoes, André Stork, and Dieter Fellner. Efficient gpu data structures and methods to solve sparse linear systems in dynamics applications. *Computer Graphics Forum*, pages no–no, 2012.

[WDW13] Jun Wu, Christian Dick, and Rüdiger Westermann. Efficient collision detection for composite finite element simulation of cuts in deformable bodies. *The Visual Computer*, 29(6-8):739–749, 2013.

[WHM09] A. Wittek, T. Hawkins, and K. Miller. On the unimportance of constitutive models in computing brain deformation for image-guided surgery. *Biomechanics and modeling in mechanobiology*, 8(1):77–84, 2009.

[Wik13] Wikipedia. Wikipedia, the free encyclopedia, 2013. [Online; accessed 22-October-2013].

[WKS+11] D. Weber, T. Kalbe, A. Stork, D. Fellner, and M. Goesele. Interactive deformable models with quadratic bases in bernstein–bézier-form. *The Visual Computer*, 27(6):473–483, 2011.

[WMKW07] A. Wittek, K. Miller, R. Kikinis, and S.K. Warfield. Patient-specific model of brain deformation: Application to medical image registration. *Journal of biomechanics*, 40(4):919–929, 2007.

[WVW+05] Ivo Wolf, Marcus Vetter, Ingmar Wegner, Thomas Böttger, Marco Nolden, Max Schöbinger, Mark Hastenteufel, Tobias Kunert, and Hans-Peter Meinzer. The medical imaging interaction toolkit. *Medical image analysis*, 9(6):594–604, 2005.

[YC06] Ziv Yaniv and Kevin Cleary. Image-guided procedures: A review. *Computer Aided Interventions and Medical Robotics*, 3, 2006.

[YM92] Chen Yang and Gérard Medioni. Object modelling by registration of multiple range images. *Image and vision computing*, 10(3):145–155, 1992.

[ZSCO+08] H. Zhang, A. Sheffer, D. Cohen-Or, Q. Zhou, O. Van Kaick, and A. Tagliasacchi. Deformation-driven shape correspondence. In *Computer Graphics Forum*, volume 27, pages 1431–1439. Wiley Online Library, 2008.

[ZSTB10] Y. Zhu, E. Sifakis, J. Teran, and A. Brandt. An efficient multigrid method for the simulation of high-resolution elastic solids. *ACM Transactions on Graphics (TOG)*, 29(2):16, 2010.

[ZT77] Olgierd Cecil Zienkiewicz and Robert Leroy Taylor. *The finite element method*, volume 3. McGraw-hill London, 1977.